Isn't It **Wonderful** When Patients Say 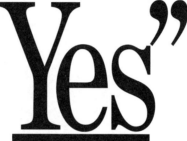 " **Yes** "

Case Acceptance for **Complete Dentistry**

Dr. Paul Homoly

Isn't It **Wonderful** When Patients Say " **Yes** "

Case Acceptance for **Complete Dentistry**

Dr. Paul Homoly

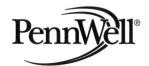

First printing 2001

ISBN
LCCN

Cover design by gary hixson
Text design by Leigh Capps Stalcup

Dedication

This book is dedicated to the many dentists and team members who have been my constant teachers of the lessons of practice and personal development.

Acknowledgements

Writing a book is like having a baby; it takes more than one to do it, they're many surprises along the way, and you're not totally sure how things will turn out. I'm pleased with this baby—you will be, too!

My first acknowledgement and thanks goes to Lisa Wiseman, my assistant for 9 years. Lisa's talent, sense of humor, and charm is a big part of the energy that runs our business, serves our clients, and makes our work fun.

My editors Virginia McCullough, Constance Holloway, and Ken Allen, and designers gary hixson, Leigh Capps Stalcup, and

Tim Breiding all helped give this book its smooth read and delightful look.

Special thanks goes to Dr. James Pride and Dr. Mark Davis for their support and advice. Their influence runs throughout this book.

Thank you to friends and supporters—Bob Salvin, Linda Miles, Kathleen Hessert, Jeffrey Gitomer—who have cheered this project on.

A big high-five to the team I work with in Charlotte—Tim Breiding, Tamara Easter, and Nikki Hrdlick. They are the ones who had to put up with the labor pains of this book!

And, of course, I'd like to thank my family—my wife Carolyn and my two wonderful and sometimes obedient children, Adam and Kristen.

Contents

CHAPTER 1

Isn't It WONDERFUL When Patients Say "Yes"

Case Acceptance for Complete Dentistry

One day I received a telephone call from Terry, a general dentist I'd known for years. He asked me to look at his practice and make some recommendations. I flew in and on the ride from the airport, we began to talk about case acceptance.

"I don't have a problem with case acceptance," Terry said. "I tell patients what they need and they generally take my recommendations."

"You mean, you just recite a list of the work they need and they say 'yes'?" I asked.

"That's right," Terry said as he smiled.

I wasn't so sure. In fact, I figured I wasn't getting the whole story, so I pressed the issue.

"How many cases do you sell that are over 3500 dollars?" I asked.

The smile disappeared from Terry's face.

I decided to persist. "How many cases do you do that you restore half or more of the teeth?"

"Listen, those kinds of patients aren't in my practice," Terry said. "I live in a conservative area and people will do what their insurance pays for, and not much more."

"Well, then, I'd say you do have a problem with case acceptance. Your problem starts where the insurance coverage ends."

"I don't do many cases much beyond what the insurance will pay for. It's almost as if there is an invisible ceiling over my patients' heads and they won't break through it, no matter how much they need the work. The way I see it, dental insurance companies are persuading the patients not to go ahead with big cases," Terry concluded.

Terry is "lucky." He's found someone to blame for his case acceptance problems—the insurance companies. Terry and thousands of dentists just like him can now enjoy gigantic gripe sessions about insurance companies. Misery loves company. If you want to stay in that mode, this book is not for you. If you want to change your attitudes and look at a new approach to case acceptance, stick with me, because you can learn what you need to know here.

All our lives we've been told: *"Don't try to sell it 'til you get it on the shelf."* Too many of us spend our careers "getting it on the shelf," so to speak. But our shelves are full. We know how to fix teeth. What we need today is information about "taking it off the shelf" by increasing acceptance for complete dentistry.

Robert's story is different from Terry's, but it has the same frustrating ending. Robert is a general dentist who has been to the mountaintop of continuing education. He has studied under all of the modern masters of our profession and has soaked up the philosophy that *"Quality dentistry sells itself."*

"I've tried to limit my practice to advanced restorative and cosmetic dentistry," Robert told me. "I pictured myself sitting at the chair doing nothing but comprehensive care, but it hasn't happened and I'm beginning to think it never will. I must be doing something wrong."

Unlike Terry, Robert blames himself for his case acceptance problems. He sees his inability to sell complete care as a personal failure and logically believes the teachers are right, and their way is the right way. He's not getting the results his teachers promised, so he believes that must be because he's not practicing the "quality dentistry" the teachers proposed. Robert's self-esteem has crashed, and so has his practice.

> **The overwhelming experience— belief—of dentists nationwide is that money is the reason patients do not accept comprehensive care.**

Terry and Robert are typical of hundreds of dentists I talk with about case acceptance. In 1996 I wrote *Dentists: An Endangered Species—A Survival Guide for Fee-for-Service Dentistry*, which explains in detail why knowing how to sell comprehensive dentistry creates great leverage in maintaining a fee-for-service practice. Since *Endangered Species* was released, I've worked with hundreds of practitioners nationwide, and I've had conversations with these men and women about case acceptance.

The consensus is that it is easy to sell simple tooth dentistry, defined as one or two appointment cosmetic procedures, accelerated endodontic procedures, and air abrasion with direct tooth colored fillings. A corollary belief states that complete dentistry is more difficult to sell. Advanced restorative and implant dentistry, cosmetic, TMJ rehabilitations, and orthodontic-orthoganthic procedures have fees attached that make most patients balk.

The dentists who do comprehensive care are those who can sell it. That sounds obvious, doesn't it? But this is not what dentists learn how to do. Attend any dental society meeting at any level and what do 99 percent of the speakers discuss? How to fix teeth. The same is true in our professional literature and dental school education. As a profession we collectively believe that the way to sell complete care is through our *technical ability* to produce quality results. The fact is, we've got it backward. *The way to produce quality is through our ability to sell complete dentistry. You will never become good and efficient at comprehensive care if you don't do it regularly.*

Complete Dentistry

The best definition I know of complete dentistry comes from Dr. Mark Davis of Clearwater, Florida. He says:

"Complete dentistry is the ability to recognize and provide as little or as much dentistry required to meet patients' needs. The

complete dentist knows how to offer a little or a lot of care with equal grace and skill."

I like Mark's definition of complete dentistry because it speaks with "equal grace" about the attitude of the dentist and the needs of the patient.

Complete dentistry includes the clinical and behavioral needs of a patient. Clinical needs relate to preventing and treating disease processes, but also include addressing aesthetic needs. Behavioral components of complete dentistry include patients' emotional concerns, their financial capacity, their relationship with your treatment team, and communication skills. Complete dentistry that does not recognize and address behavioral issues is not complete dentistry at all. In the language of the day, it's "an accident waiting to happen."

Although this book emphasizes case acceptance for rehabilitative care, there's much to be said for offering minimal care in some circumstances. To again quote Mark Davis: *"When you recommend, for good reasons, that patients not rebuild their mouth, you'll discover that they recognize your professionalism and often become some of your best referring patients. Young dentists miss this point."*

The dentistry is only part of the patient's experience. Complete dentists treat the mouth and the mind. **Dr. Mark Davis**

The Business of Selling

Throughout this book you will see references to "selling," "high-fee," and "low-fee." *Don't misinterpret my language and infer from my words that I advocate squeezing every nickel out of your patients.* I realize that some readers may interpret the language of selling as being too retail, too anti-establishment, even too aggressive and "in your face," and might leave the impression that I have a cash register where my heart is supposed to be. This isn't true. I have one purpose for writing this book. *My goal is to help you gain case acceptance for complete comprehensive dentistry, not to sell things in the retail sense.* You are not a typical retailer, so you aren't selling gadgets and gizmos for their own sake.

Most dentists are good at gaining case acceptance for what I'll call tooth dentistry, that is, fixing one or two teeth at a time. This book is about case acceptance for *complete dentistry*, which I define as eliminating all the dental disease and creating optimal aesthetics. I use the words "sell" and "influence" interchangeably. When you read the phrase "sell high-fee complete dentistry," interpret it as "influencing a patient to accept treatment for the elimination and control of dental disease and optimal dental aesthetics."

Keep in mind that it's the expense, the fees associated with our care, that patients object to. Do patients object to the high quality and comprehensive nature of our care? No. They object to the fee. Yet, where do we spend the greatest energy and time? In explaining the quality and comprehensiveness of the care. But patients want care. That's why they're in your chair. It's the fee that needs to be sold. When was the last time you attended a course on how to talk about money with persuasion and impact?

Dentistry needs a new language that addresses money.

If you want your fee-for-service practice to survive, high-fee complete dentistry is in your future. Here's why: Let's call fees below 3500 dollars low-fee tooth dentistry. In this range, dental insurance has a major influence on patients. Dental insurance usually reimburses a major percentage of the fee in this low-fee tooth dentistry range. Additionally, managed care companies reimburse for low-fee tooth dentistry, which also attracts management service organizations. Low-fee tooth dentistry prevails in discount dentistry clinics, dental schools, and the military. Most of the competition in dentistry is for low-fee tooth dentistry, and all third-party intervention is in the low-fee tooth dentistry range.

The way out of being manipulated by insurance companies is to go from low-fee tooth dentistry up to high-fee complete dentistry. Insurance companies and your competitors will not follow, which means that the future of fee-for-service dentistry is in complete high-fee dentistry.

How do you know if you're a high-fee complete dentist or a low-fee tooth dentist? Answer the following questions to find out:

1. Do most of your accepted treatment plans total less than 3,500 dollars?

2. Is dental insurance reimbursement critical to your survival?

3. Do your hygiene collections, i.e., routine cleanings, represent nearly 30 to 40 percent of your total collections?

4. Are most of your appointments scheduled for sixty minutes or less?

5. Are twenty new patients a month insufficient to meet your income goals?

If you answered yes to most of the above, you have a low-fee tooth dentistry practice. Being a low-fee tooth dentist is not wrong, but you'll spend your career working harder for less return than is possible with a practice based on complete care.

My preference for complete dentistry does not result from a desire to see dentists line their pockets. However, I'm a strong advocate of offering complete dentistry, which has higher fees associated with it. Remember that fee issues, not dentistry, trigger most patient objections. Fee issues need to be communicated with influence, empathy, and confidence.

Much of this book is about fee issues. I know you love dentistry or you wouldn't be reading this book. When you know how to handle the language of fees *and* provide more complete dentistry, you'll love dentistry more. That's the goal of this book.

Stages of Practice

Your style and process of case acceptance largely depends on where you are in your career. If you're in the first decade of practice, you need to prove yourself. You focus on building your skills, increasing efficiency and productivity, and surviving. During this phase you focus on issues revolving around you. When it comes to case acceptance for complete care, the early stage is the most difficult.

When you're in the second decade of practice, case acceptance for complete care improves. Patients you've treated refer their friends. The number of patients you have in your re-care system grows. Overall you begin to see more new patients who know you or know about you; these patients are in your office because you offer the type of dentistry they want and they have the financial capacity to pay for it. In real estate and other sales settings, individuals who know what they want and have the means to pay for it are called "qualified buyers." In your second decade of practice, you'll begin to see more "qualified patients" and as a result, case acceptance naturally improves. When this happens, you can shift your focus away from yourself and focus on clinical quality and professional growth.

Dentists in their third decade see many "qualified patients." Among new patients many have considered having their teeth fixed for years, and during those years they've heard the names of the same dentists come up again and again. When these patients are ready they come in, and with very little persuasion they accept complete care. Dentists in their third decade focus on relationships with patients, staff, other dentists, and with the wider community of professionals and the lay public.

**As you and your practice mature,
your case acceptance style
will evolve.**

    This book is intended as a guide, rather than a specific recipe for "the one right way to do it." Whether you're in the first, second, or third decade of practice, this book has value for you.

Coming Attractions

    All the concepts presented in this book work together to form a unified program for selling complete care dentistry. Each component is a building block that strengthens your understanding of the process. We start with the philosophy that forms the foundation of this program for complete care dentistry, and then we move on to a discussion of communication skills and the way they integrate into the recommended structure of the program. Early chapters answer the "why" questions before we move on to examine the skills that show you "how" to implement the program. Information about structure shows you "where," "to whom," and "when" to apply this philosophy.

    Some material may sound familiar, while other information may be new to you, but keep in mind that the familiar and unfamiliar features are woven together to form a unique system that specifically addresses dental practice issues. You'll find that the heart of the program is found in the techniques of *StorySelling*® and in the important concept known as the *Spectrum of Appeal*™. These communication tools will take you a long way on your journey to increased acceptance of complete care dentistry and I urge you to consider them the key to implementing this program—and enriching the rest of your life as you deepen your understanding of human behavior.

Individual chapters provide practical advice about targeting patients, providing value, and understanding the difference between quality and suitability of care. We'll also explore the concept of patient readiness. One of the most frustrating experiences dentists confront is presenting a level of dental care patients are not ready to accept.

This book also introduces a practical tool I call the ***critical dialogues*** that guides you through the sequence of steps in the process of case acceptance of complete care. You will find sample dialogues that you can adapt to meet your needs. I know from my own experience and those of my clients that these dialogues are effective and have the power to maximize case acceptance.

If you're reading this book, you are probably thinking about your future and the future of dentistry. You may be frustrated with insurance companies and you want to use the technical skills you have spent years perfecting. *One of my primary goals for this book is to help you do the dentistry you love, rather than the level of dentistry you feel forced to accept.* To that end, I offer information about marketing and I explain why attracting denture patients creates demand for restorative and cosmetic procedures.

Finally, I have included some information about the dynamic I call "Mars and Venus in the Dental Office," which demonstrates the way gender differences influence the dental office environment. It is my hope that the discussion leads to greater harmony among dentists and their staff. And speaking of gender, I have added a chapter that discusses the unique opportunities women have in dentistry today and the ways they are changing the image and expectations of dentists and their practices.

Throughout this book you will find anecdotes and quotes I've gathered from dentists and team members. These examples come from individuals with typical general and specialty practices who have been through case acceptance training with me and are experiencing many real-world applications of the skills this book teaches. Their success and the success of hundreds of practitioners just like them prove that these principles work—and you can make them work for you.

Developed with this book are four other tools to boost your case acceptance for complete dentistry. Each of the five tools, including this book, is designed as a learning system. I'd recommend that you use this system in the following sequence.

1. Read the book. I've provided wide margins for note taking, comments, and questions. It's a good idea to give key staff members their own copy of this book.

2. Access my web site, www.paulhomoly.com, for information previously published. I've indicated in the book when the web site should be accessed. My web site offers learning tools updates and new insights into the process of case acceptance.

3. Watch the video presentation. The video is an excellent visual communication tool that best describes a central element of case acceptance, the Spectrum of Appeal. Although the Spectrum of Appeal is discussed in the book and audio program, the video program offers the most clarity into this process. The video presentation is a great tool to use at staff meetings.

4. Listen to the audio program. The audio program is designed to reinforce the critical dialogs of case acceptance. Listen to the audio program several times while driving. You'll learn the dialogs just like you learn the words of songs when you listen to them many times.

5. Participate in Case Acceptance Coaching. Coaching is designed to support you and your team in the new concepts and skills of case acceptance. There is no substitute for coaching. I see much greater behavioral and communication competencies in teams who have been coached than in teams who have only read and listened to this information. The book, audio program, video presentation, and web site all are designed to be prerequisite materials for the coaching. They provide information, the coaching creates the skills.

I hope you will return to this book many times, and work with the material until you know it well. Because the information is organized as a course in case acceptance for complete dentistry, it's best read from beginning to end, because each chapter builds on the previous one. Enjoy!

CHAPTER 2

WHO'S
Wrong With Me
Today?

Communication Skills, Philosophy & Structure of Case Acceptance for Complete Dentistry

Are you upset when patients say no? Does it drive you nuts when they call to ask you to send their records to the dentist across the street? Before you let these annoying situations take over your psyche, recognize that for many dentists, it's not a question of "What's wrong with me today?" but "Who's wrong with me today?" If you're frustrated by low case acceptance for complete dentistry, it may be time to look in the mirror. Blaming patients for refusing your care is like shooting the messenger. Stop looking at who's refusing your care and start looking at who's presenting it.

Janet is a top-notch restorative and cosmetic dentist. She's been in practice fifteen years in a competitive urban area. She's experienced significant success in her career, enjoying collections in the 600,000-dollar to the 750,000-dollar range. However in the last few years she's seen her practice decline.

"Years ago I knew I had it made," she told me. "Patients accepted comprehensive care, which in my practice meant six to twelve veneers and multiple crowns. Today, my biggest cases are two and three teeth!"

"Have you read my book?" I asked.

"Yes, I have and I do it exactly as you say, but it hasn't helped," she said.

Our conversation ended with her disappointed—and disappointing—statement, but a few months later I held a seminar in Janet's area. Later, over dinner, we discussed her practice again.

"Let's say I'm a new patient," I said, "and I call your office and ask to get my teeth cleaned. How do you handle this?"

"Well, first of all, I don't let the patient give me the diagnosis and treatment plan over the telephone," she replied. "I don't run my practice by scheduling appointments with new patients just for cleanings. All new patients receive a comprehensive examination, and based on our findings, I recommend care. We explain our standards and patients are asked to rise to meet those standards." Janet's tone exuded pride and certainty.

Janet had several other "standards" she insisted on maintaining, which included not accepting insurance payments, rigorous oral hygiene procedures, and thorough patient education. All her standards sounded correct, as if they were the right things to do, but it took only a few minutes to see that she had some rigid ways of doing business. Her rigid philosophy was driving patients from her practice and she blamed the patients, the community, and other dentists for her decline. But who is wrong with Janet today?

As we spoke I noticed that Janet did not maintain eye contact with me. She looked away as she spoke, and her voice was flat and expressionless as she "issued" her complaints. She didn't smile as her answers to my questions ran on and on. She had excellent command of language, but her overall communication style resembled that of a lecturer.

When I asked Janet about the structure of her case acceptance process, she adopted the method I described in my book, *Dentists: An Endangered Species*. However, Janet has successfully implemented only one-third of the process necessary for patients to accept complete dentistry. The structure represents just a portion of what is needed; Janet has missed the philosophy and the communication/leadership skills, and relies on the structure to carry the day. When dentists tell me they are not experiencing success with selling complete dentistry, that sends a signal that tells that, like Janet, they're missing one or more parts of the three-part process of selling high-fee dentistry: communication skills, philosophy, and structure.

Communication Skills

What are the differences between a dentist with great clinical skills who is nearly broke, and one with average clinical skills who is rich? *Personality*. We express our personality through our language and leadership qualities. Unfortunately many dentists don't put language and developing leadership ability on their continuing education dance card.

Have you ever met someone you've immediately liked or disliked? No doubt you have. Remember that your complete care patients have had the same experience with you and your staff.

I remember a conversation I had years ago with my administrative assistant, Tamara. She said: "Doc, you never open up to any of us. You don't care about so many of the things we do. The only way we know what you're thinking is by the look on your face."

"I *do* care a lot about what goes on with you and the rest of the staff," I said. "I don't talk to you about your personal lives because I respect your privacy. The way I see it, if you had a problem you'll tell me."

"I do have a problem."

"What is it?"

"You don't talk to us."

We're judged by how we express ourselves. We do not show respect by withholding effective expression, nor is this kind of communication style a signal of high intelligence.

The conversation with Tamara provided insight into communication with patients. In general, *low-fee tooth dentistry patients put a low premium on the expressiveness of their dentist; complete care patients place high emphasis on expressiveness and they need to connect with you.* If you're not expressing yourself, patients will not accept your dentistry.

Ask most dentists if they've had training in communication skills and they likely will say yes. They may describe a personality classification system that outlines four basic personality types or they may have knowledge of other ways to describe personality types. These personality systems are useful as a foundation, and they help us with the art of communication. The tools we need to sell complete dentistry are more related to the ability to express ourselves than they are to profiling personality types. While I am not against expanding our knowledge of human behavior and personality, I am against relying on them as the sole solution to selling complete dentistry.

Developing communication skills makes us more expressive, and expressiveness makes your ideas and recommendations more interesting, memorable, and persuasive. This book organizes communication skills into three parts:

1. **The Spectrum of Appeal**™
2. **Tools of Expression**
3. **StorySelling**®

Think of these three components as the "communication package" that connects you with your patients. Selling low-fee tooth dentistry is about selling procedures. A patient may say yes to a crown or two from a dentist with no personality, but *selling complete dentistry is about selling yourself.*

Philosophy

The philosophy of selling complete high-fee dentistry is different from low-fee tooth dentistry. The rules for tooth dentistry include: Inform before you perform, educate the patient, emphasize prevention, and use technical explanations.

Complete dentistry has different rules, which are best understood by looking at four distinct parts:
- Focus on target patients.
- Build value early.
- Know the difference between quality and suitability.
- Understand why raising patients' dental IQ may not make them ready for care.

The rules for low-fee tooth dentistry will not work with high-fee complete care because patient behaviors and expectations at the high-fee complete care level are different from those at the low-fee tooth dentistry level.

Let's say you're flying an airplane at 10,000 feet. You pull back on the yoke and the airplane climbs. You push forward and you dive. Turn the yoke to the right and you roll right. Very predictable. Now let's say we put your airplane in the space shuttle and blast you to 500,000 feet, 94 miles into the vacuum of space. Then we open the shuttle doors and drop you out. You pull back on the yoke and guess what? Nothing happens. Push forward, roll right? Same thing, nothing happens. Why? At high altitudes the rules are different. The rules of aerodynamics change at high altitudes. The rules of case acceptance change at high altitudes—the high-fee levels.

What worked at 10,000 feet doesn't work at 500,000 feet. The laws of aerodynamics at high altitudes are not linear extensions of low altitudes. Even by making the wings bigger and having a stronger engine, it won't fly at 500,000 feet. Likewise, what works at the 500-dollar level doesn't work at the 10,000-plus dollar level. Longer preclinical interviews, more in-depth clinical examinations, stricter home care standards, increased high-

tech patient education, exhaustive informed consent procedures, and more elaborate visual aids do not represent what
makes high-fee complete care cases fly.

Relationship skills make complete care cases fly. At the high-
fee complete care level, patients are buying the relationship with
you as much as they are buying the dentistry. The rules for developing relationships are different from the rules that guide your
clinical skills. You already know the clinical skills; now it's time
to complete your education by learning relationship skills.
Throughout this book, we'll examine each component of these
philosophies and help you practice dentistry at high altitudes.

Structure

The *structure* of case acceptance for complete dentistry
includes the sequence of steps with which you move patients
through the process from their initial telephone call to the
beginning of care.

The structure has six steps:
- Initial experience
- Diagnostic records
- Case preview
- Case discussion
- Case discussion letter
- Preoperative appointment

These steps are not necessarily completed in six appointments; under some circumstances, the entire process can be
completed in two appointments, although it is most commonly
completed in three.

In the team approach, defined as the general dentist and specialist working together to sell complete dentistry, the structure includes seven steps:
- Initial appointment–General dentist
- Diagnostic records–General dentist
- Case Preview–General dentist
- Case Discussion–General dentist
- Referral to specialist–Specialty diagnosis and treatment plan
- Case Discussion Letter–GP and Specialist
- Preoperative appointment–GP and Specialist

The Five Critical Dialogues

Embroidered throughout the structure are five critical dialogues. I've learned that the weakest link my clients and readers have when implementing this case acceptance process is mastery of five critical dialogues. To master these dialogues you must use the information outlined in the chapters on philosophy and communication/leadership skills.

I've labeled the critical dialogues CD-1, CD-2, and so forth. Briefly, they are defined in the following ways:

CD-1: Identifying and scheduling the target patient.

CD-2: Offering a choice between the lifetime strategy of dental care versus treating the patient's chief complaint.

CD-3: Introducing the concept of dental budget.

CD-4: Previewing the treatment plan in the future tense—case preview.

CD-5: Determining the budget.

What follows is an overview of each critical dialogue to give you a sense of the content and the sequence of the entire structure. In succeeding chapters, each is examined in greater detail.

Critical Dialogue Number One (CD-1):
Identifying and schedule the target patient.
You'll learn the concept of the ***compelled target patient***. These patients want and need the dentistry you love to do. This dialogue occurs over the telephone between the new patient and the scheduler.

Critical Dialogue Number Two (CD-2):
Lifetime versus chief complaint strategy.
CD-2 occurs during a first appointment, immediately after a simple initial examination is completed. In CD-2 the dentist asks: "Are you interested in having your chief complaint fixed, or are you interested in pursuing a lifetime strategy of dental health?" Another good way of asking this is: "Are you interested in having your chief complaint fixed, or are you interested in fixing all of your teeth. What's best for you now?"
This question guides us to the route of the most appropriate care for this patient and demonstrates that we're willing to provide great service. The question also helps reduce our frustration and wasted time by eliminating the detailed compre-

hensive examination and consultation on people who are neither interested nor ready for what we offer.

Keep in mind that we need to prove ourselves to new patients. Sometimes it's best to fix a sore spot on a denture, make a temporary crown, or extract a sore tooth to assure patients that they are in the right place. Let them experience your care, skill, and judgment before you ask if they're ready for a lifetime strategy. CD-2 tells patients that they can proceed with care on their schedule.

Critical Dialogue Number Three:
Introducing the concept of the dental budget.

CD-3 is for patients who choose to pursue a lifetime strategy of dental health, which means having all their teeth fixed. This dialogue between the dentist and the patient takes the form of questions: "I'm really good about staying within a budget if I know I need to. Have you given any thought to your budget?"

This dialogue is not designed to prompt your patients to tell you what their budgets are, but rather to foreshadow a discussion about the level of dental care that fits their budgets and schedules.

This may be a new concept for you. You may think that talking about money is a great idea; on the other hand, some of you may want to burn this book. But before you toss it on the flames, give these ideas a chance to develop. Your patients will thank you.

Critical Dialogue Number Four:
Previewing the treatment plan.

In CD-4 the dentist speaks in the future tense. CD-4 informs the patients of what's possible but stops short of carving that recommendation in stone. For example, during CD-4 you may say: "A good way to make your front teeth beautiful is to fuse a thin enamel colored coating over them. They're called laminate veneers and when you're ready, and it fits within your budget, that would be a good way to go." CD-4 hints at treatment recommendations.

Critical Dialogue Number Five:
Determining the budget.

CD-5 takes place after the patient has an idea of what's possible (you informed the patient about this in CD-4) but is not yet fully aware of its cost. CD-5 takes the form of a reminder from the dentist: "Last time I recommended that you think about your dental budget. Give me an idea what you're comfortable with and I'll guarantee that I'll design your care to fit within that budget." CD-5 reveals the possibility of balancing your dentistry with their budget. The dentistry they need that doesn't fall within the budget is planned for succeeding years. The principle? *Do not dilute the quality or comprehensiveness of the treatment plan, but implement the best plan over time.*

In succeeding chapters, I'll discuss the six/seven step structure of case acceptance for complete dentistry and show how the five critical dialogues fit within them. It's tempting to think that one right way exists to do case acceptance and then repeat the exact process every time. Throw out that thinking right away. Case acceptance is not a one-size-fits-all process.

There is no one right way of doing things. You are not creating a rigid system in which everyone in your practice goes through the same process for case acceptance.

Rigid systems are popular because they are easy and predictable. Every patient gets a preclinical interview; every patient gets a complete examination; every patient gets full-mouth radiographs; every patient watches the videotape on periodontal disease; and so forth. The "every patient" approach helps organize the process and works well at the low-fee tooth dentistry level. At the complete dentistry level, however, the "every patient" approach can fail because it doesn't make distinctions between patients.

Is your case acceptance system for a young male patient who needs a few fillings and wants his teeth cleaned (tooth dentistry) the same as for a sixty-year-old female with a failing full-mouth reconstruction (complete dentistry)? If it is, then two things are happening in your practice. First, you're making the tooth dentistry patients angry about too many radiographs, too many appointments, lack of insurance coverage, and not getting what they came for. Second, you're frustrating your complete care patients by overanalyzing/educating, overselling, not listening to them, and not taking yes for an answer.

Have you ever learned ballroom dancing on a cruise ship? It's easy. They paint the foot pattern of the dance on the floor, and all you do is stay in tempo and follow the pattern. It's a system that works at the beginner level.

But what if the band changes its tune from a waltz to a rumba while you're still following the painted waltz foot pattern? You're not going to be able to dance. The only way you can dance if you're locked into your pattern is to ask the band to change its tune and that's not going to happen.

If you have the steps of case acceptance painted on the floor and you know only one dance—"The Waltz of the New Patient"—and that complete care patient comes in whistling a different tune, you're going to be dancing with your staff. And will your complete care patients change their tune for you? That's not going to happen either.

Case acceptance for complete dentistry is not a puzzle to solve. It's a dance that calls for you to interpret the music of the patient. If you want better case acceptance for complete dentistry take the focus off changing the patient, and change yourself by adopting a new philosophy and structure for case acceptance of complete dentistry. Learn the tools of expressiveness to make your ideas and recommendations more interesting, memorable, and persuasive.

CHAPTER 3

Dentistry: It's
EASIER DONE
Than
Said

Complete Dentistry
Communication Skills

Dentists own a strong societal stereotype: dullness. We have our own category of jokes, just like "dumb blondes" and "drunk Irishmen." We know we are far from dull, but most of us admit we sound that way. The fact is, communication is a *learned* skill, but our education has not prepared us to effectively communicate in the various roles we fill in order to succeed: leadership, management, sales, motivation, instruction, mentoring, and coaching. For many of us, dentistry is easier to *do* than it is to talk about. However, if you want to sell complete dentistry, you must learn to engage in effective communication, which by definition is never dull.

Language is a practice-building tool we too often overlook. Like the fingers on our hands, we take our language for granted. Our ability to express ourselves may become lost in the maze of facts and processes of our dentistry. Like pocket change we toss into a drawer, we forget about the importance of our language and in the process our words are devalued. If you want to sell complete dentistry, then your language must be memorable, persuasive, and inspiring. So when we ask, "Why the "dull dentist" stereotypes?" the answer involves the inability to express to our patients and staff who we are, what we love, and how we feel about what we do.

Complete care patients want to know who you are, what you love, and how you feel about what you do.

Language Atrophy

In dentistry our language has atrophied. It has contracted under the pressure of information and technology. We've created a world of abbreviations and jargon: URLs, CD-ROMs, MODs, emergence contours, and osseointegration. We are more capable of reciting the facts from our practice brochure or a dry rendition of our mission statement than we are of telling a simple, lively story that illustrates who we are, what we do, and why we do it.

While attending the Chicago Midwinter Dental Meeting I bumped into two old buddies, Joe and Steve, with whom I attended dental school. We shared a joyous, backslapping reunion and then we sat and talked.

"So, Joe," I asked, "how's dentistry treating you?"

"Good, I guess," he said casually.

I was waiting for some details of why it was good, but they weren't forthcoming.

"So, Steve, have you seen many of the guys we went through school with?" I asked, hoping to hear some stories.

"No, I haven't seen many."

I decided to try again. "So what's new with you guys? What are you excited about?"

A scrap of energy finally made its way into the conversation, but I couldn't help but notice my friends' flat, almost monotonous speech pattern, not unlike what I hear in so many dentists. This is strange, I thought. I remembered Joe and Steve as being expressive and alive.

Over the years, my two friends had created successful careers and they weren't unhappy with dentistry. But I wouldn't have known that from the tone of their voices or their facial expressions. I wondered if years of maintaining that flat professional tone of voice when speaking to patients had contaminated their ability to communicate and left them with this narrow and, frankly, dull range of expression.

Is this trend unique to dentistry? Not at all. I've noticed the same lack of expressiveness when I work with engineers or people in the financial services industry. It seems the higher we go in professional education, the more specialized and abstract our language becomes. We withhold expressiveness out of fear that it interferes or competes with our credibility. But I guarantee you that *no one ever lost credibility by being interesting.*

Are Dentists Just Introverts?

Maybe you've heard that dentists are introverts who prefer quiet offices to large gatherings. I hear this analysis used as an excuse when I talk to groups about the lack of expansive language and expression among dentists. I always challenge this assumption and ask you to remember the students with whom you went through dental school. How many of them were introverts? How many had flat, serious facial expressions? How many of them were quiet and shy?

We had 103 students in the University of Illinois 1975 graduating class and I don't remember the majority of them being introverts. The people I went to dental school with drank beer and raised hell! We needed cages. The serious and shy behavior labeled introversion is actually learned in dental school and, most significantly, is "perfected" in the postgraduate continuing education process.

Introversion is learned in dental school and "perfected" during the postgraduate continuing education process.

Lessons in Poor Communication

Consider the typical continuing education course. First, the courses are labeled as lectures, which implies that the speaker will do the talking and we'll do the listening. Listening is quiet behavior. Next, the lectures are given by authority figures who over time reach celebrity status in dentistry. Our culture emulates celebrities. So as celebrity authority figures/speakers present their lectures we admire and model this behavior.

How do most speakers present their material? They are literally in the dark. They show slides as they lecture and generally do not make eye contact with their audience. Since no one can see them, they deliver their lectures without facial animation and expression. With a serious tone, these lecturers deliver information in a serious technical fashion, with an emphasis on processes and procedures.

As attendees in these continuing education lectures, what do we learn? We inadvertently learn to be introverted. We learn to communicate without making eye contact, and just like these authority figures, we come to associate minimal facial expressions and a serious, analytical tone with significance and even celebrity status. Is this introversion? I don't think so. I believe it's a poor communication style we unconsciously learned during continuing education programs. These authority figures did not set out to turn us into men and women with stilted communication styles. It happened inadvertently.

Just as you can learn great communication skills by listening to great communicators, you can learn poor communication skills from poor communicators. That's exactly what's happened in dentistry.

Since great communication skills have never been a high priority skill for dentists, we easily forgive the brilliant clinician who presents excellent visual and technical information in a flat and lifeless manner. Most of the continuing education speakers are not speakers at all. What they call speaking is actually narrating their visual aids. I'm not saying this is wrong; I'm saying it's incomplete.

Content desperately needs expressiveness to make it interesting and memorable. Most CE programs are organized and rehearsed with the focus on slides and audiovisual aids. Have you ever suffered through multiple all-day slide shows? How empowered and alive do you feel after that?

The Bad News First

The bad news is that the collapse of language yields the lifeless and abstract communication we call jargon. Using jargon to communicate with other dentists is fine, but use it with complete-care patients and you'll lose their interest and even their sense of confidence in you. Many dentists use jargon unconsciously. Without thinking, they talk to patients about restorations, tooth reduction, anatomy, contours, Empress, osseointergration, parathesia, and so on. Jargon is a kind of dialect—you don't know you speak in dialect until you hear someone who doesn't.

The good news is you can stop this language free fall and rediscover the colorful, spirited, and visual language you once had. I know you had it. You've just forgotten it or haven't given yourself permission to use it.

Now the Good News

Remember that little tune you sang in first grade, the alphabet song: "A, B, C, D, E, F, G…" (sung to the tune of "Twinkle, Twinkle Little Star")? Isn't it amazing that you still remember it? The reason you can pass the song on to your children is that the information you learned, the alphabet, is embroidered into a little melody that's fun to sing. Information plus fun equals learning. Colorful, spirited, and visual language is easy to remember. The language of case acceptance for complete dentistry needs to be easy to remember.

Information + Fun = Learning

A Lifetime of Learning

We now have a whole generation of individuals who have grown up with the computer. So, how did the twenty-eight-year-old, who now writes complex computer language for Microsoft, bond with the computer? By playing games, by having fun with the computer. Remember Asteroid and PAC Man games? They were the fun activities that anchored the learning, which has led to the technology that runs our world. I'm convinced that when the fun stops, the learning stops. Maybe not all learning but certainly learning that is effortless and lasts a lifetime. *Information plus fun equals learning.*

What People Remember Most

The next chapters focus on communication, and I'm going to teach you to be memorable and persuasive through the use of language. Keep in mind that the purpose of this material on communication is to help promote case acceptance. No communication or sales technique will sell complete care every time. Not everyone will say yes to you, but if you are memorable and persuasive, they'll never forget that you offered. And over the long term, what is remembered is sold.

CHAPTER 4

People WHO LIKE YOU Can Justify Anything

The Spectrum of Appeal™

Consider all the people you've listened to over the course of your life: teachers, salespeople, co-workers, politicians, managers, vendors, clergy, bankers, physicians, dentists, and friends. Of the thousands of people you've heard speak, how many of them are truly outstanding speakers? When I pose this question to men and women in my seminars most tell me that they can think of very few who reached that level, usually fewer than five.

The number is so small because most speakers lack an emotional connection with their audiences because they fail to blend emotional appeal into their language.

Your job is to embroider emotional appeal into the language of case acceptance because people buy based on emotion and justify their decision with facts. And patients who like you can justify anything.

A person usually has two reasons for doing something. One that sounds good, and the real reason.

J.P. Morgan

In dentistry we are strongly biased in favor of the facts. This is fine. Facts are good; they help us make the right diagnosis and recommendations for care. However patients don't rely exclusively on facts to make up their mind. They use emotion, and lots of it.

Complete-care patients have two reasons for accepting your care. One that sounds good: They need the dentistry; and the real reason, an emotional one: They like and trust you.

The Spectrum of Appeal

An easy tool exists to help you begin embroidering emotional appeal into your language. It's called the Spectrum of Appeal and is a visual representation, a pattern showing the way great speakers create broad appeal blending logic and emotion. (See figure 1.)

As you can see, the Spectrum of Appeal is a graph that represents the type and intensity of appeal. **The vertical axis represents appeal**: logical appeal above the gray line, emotional

FIGURE 1: The Spectrum of Appeal

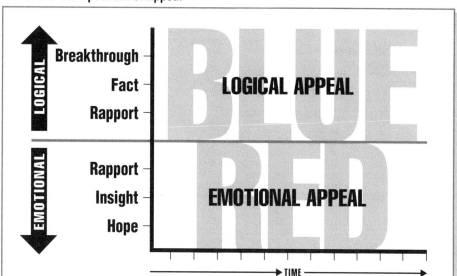

below. As you move up the logic line, the logical appeal increases. As you move down the emotional line, the emotional appeal increases. The gray line represents neutral appeal. **The horizontal axis represents sequential time**, the time between the beginning and end of your communication.

We Start with Rapport

The first order of logical appeal is rapport. When you establish similarity, agreement, and harmony you establish rapport. Establish rapport in the logical spectrum by introducing rational statements about yourself: name, location, history, occupation, role, age, and so forth. These statements establish common bonds with your listeners, hence creating a similarity and likability between the two of you. You may be similar to your patients in education, occupation, where they live, what they need from you, and how you can meet their needs.

████████████████████

You don't build rapport by talking about your mission statement, state-of-the-art dental remedies, or by sticking the patients in front of a video monitor and having them watch a video on periodontal disease.

If I were to build rapport with a patient in the logical spectrum it might sound like this:

"Hello, I'm Dr. Paul Homoly. I've practiced dentistry for twenty years here in Charlotte. I live in Charlotte with my wife Carolyn and my two kids Adam and Kristen. I help patients who have severe problems caused by missing teeth."

Just the Facts

The next higher level of logical appeal includes facts: ideas, data, and information. Facts are the most common level of the logical spectrum. This was Sargent Dick Friday's favorite form of logic, "Just the facts, ma'am." It's at this level that patient education, consent, home care instructions, explanations of procedures, and so forth, takes place.

Ah-ha—the Breakthrough

The highest order of logical appeal is breakthrough. A breakthrough is an "ah-ha!" experience, which occurs when the listener understands and sees new relationships among the facts, figures, ideas, and other data. *Breakthroughs take us beyond the facts.* Breakthroughs are the biggest truths, realized when we see ideas strung together like pearls on a necklace. We no longer see the individual pearls, we see their combined beauty. Einstein's famous formula E=MC2 is a breakthrough. For dentists, mastering occlusion, aesthetics, and biomechanics are examples of breakthroughs that string many facts together.

I experienced a breakthrough twenty years ago when I was attending the Pankey Institute. It was 6:30 in the evening, and I was struggling with an equilibration exercise on a plastic mannequin. Dr. John Anderson strolled up and leaned over to watch me work.

"Do you mind if I show you a few things?" he asked. What happened in the next thirty minutes was the purest, clearest teaching I ever experienced. That day I achieved a breakthrough in my understanding of occlusion and equilibration.

Building Emotional Rapport

The emotional spectrum also has levels of intensity. The first level of emotional appeal is rapport, and just like logical appeal, rapport in the emotional spectrum fosters familiarity, similarity, and likability. For example, if I were to build rapport in the emotional spectrum with a professional dental audience it might sound like this:

> *"Hello, I'm Paul Homoly, and for the last twenty years I've had the privilege of helping patients who found themselves on the top of the junk pile of dental cripples. My work has been very fulfilling because it helped relieve the most common crippling dental disability—total edentulism—and actually changed people's lives."*

Notice the differences in building rapport in the logical and emotional spectrum. Logical rapport addresses the issues of how, what, when, and how many. Emotional rapport focuses on reasons and is more visual in its language than logical rapport. Emotional rapport includes expected, familiar, and comfortable emotions.

Gaining Insight

The next level of emotional appeal is insight, which is an understanding or perception of things. Insights reflect how we feel about the facts, and may include unexpected, unfamiliar, and uncomfortable emotions or realizations. Typical examples of emotions at this level are: surprise, humor, sorrow, conflict, fear, frustration, passion, depression, love, hate, excitement, boredom, greed, generosity, envy, and respect. Emotions that are *opposites*, like happiness and sorrow, are found *together* in this spectrum. This level does not qualify the emotion as desirable or undesirable, but organizes them based on their effect on us.

Optimism: Hope in Action

The deepest level of emotional appeal is hope. Hope is and always has been the deepest, most fundamental motivating emotion. The optimistic—hope-filled—person thrives emotionally. Without hope, there is no life. You have a wonderful opportunity to bring hope to your patients. Hope is the ultimate benefit of dental health care.

Red and Blue Spectrum

To make the Spectrum of Appeal more visual, I'm going to call the logical spectrum the blue spectrum and emotional the red spectrum: *logic = blue, emotion = red.*

What blue spectrum tools do we use in the dental office? What appeals to the patient's logic? How about study models, radiographs, photographs, periodontal charting, patient education, diagnosis, treatment plans, insurance forms, technical explanations, brochures, records, oral hygiene instruction, medical history, and on and on. In fact, just about everything we touch and see in the dental office, along with most of our conversations, are based on logical appeal. We use an abundant number of blue spectrum tools. Most of our dental school and continuing education is blue spectrum, so it's easy to see why dentists and staff use blue spectrum tools almost exclusively and are the most comfortable with it.

If a major part of appeal is emotional, what red spectrum tools do we use with the ease and consistency as our blue spectrum tools? Make a list of all the red spectrum tools you use. The list isn't as long nor does it come to mind as readily, does it? What this tells us is that if we want to optimize our appeal, then we need to recognize, develop, and use more red spectrum tools. Attitude, connection, disclosure, and visual language are red spectrum tools. (More about these in a later chapter.)

Remember: *People buy on emotion and justify with logic.* What the Spectrum of Appeal creates is a visual representation of blending logical and emotional appeal. The broadest appeal combines both logic and emotion.

Persuasion, leadership, sales, motivation, and any change in behavior or growth result from a combination of logical and emotional appeal.

Rapport: Blue and Red

Let's diagram a dialogue that blends logic and emotion. You walk into the consultation area to meet a new patient. After brief hellos, the patient says, "Tell me about your practice."

The goal of your dialogue is to build rapport so the patient can learn something about you (logical appeal) and begin to like you (emotional appeal). The logical appeal of your dialogue is shown in **bold italic** typeface; the emotional appeal in shown in *regular italics*:

> *"Mrs. Fitzpatrick, I graduated from the University of Illinois's School of Dentistry in Chicago in 1975. I spent a few years in the Navy as a dentist. I was stationed at Marine Corp Air at Cherry Point, North Carolina. That's how I ended up in North Carolina."*

"My wife wanted to raise our kids in a more relaxed environment than Chicago, so we stayed in this area. I built this building twelve years ago with the help of my brother Guy, who is a contractor and still lives in Chicago.

"Our practice specializes in implant and cosmetic dentistry. In addition to my practice, I teach advanced dental techniques nationwide. My partner, Dr. Davis, focuses on cosmetic and family dentistry and I focus on implant and permanent tooth replacements."

"Many of my patients kid me because of my Chicago accent, but they also tell me I'm a pretty good guy even though I'm a Yankee!"

"Mrs. Fitzpatrick, how can I help you today?"

Notice how the dialogue swings from logical to emotional appeal at the level of rapport (See figure 2). The logical appeal relates the facts of the therapeutic features of the practice. The emotional appeal discloses several things about me: I'm married, I'm a parent, I respect my wife's opinion, I'm from Chicago, I get along with my brother, my brother's name is Guy, and I have a sense of humor. I've told the patient a lot about me so she can relate to me in a way other than as her dentist. This relaxes her and makes me more approachable and believable. I've covered all the bases—logic and emotion—and established rapport in the process.

FIGURE 2: Alternate between logical and emotional appeal.

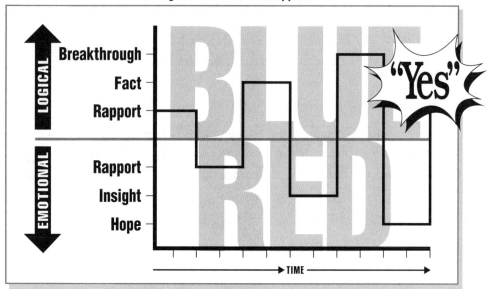

Facts and Insights

As our conversation continues, we increase the level of logical and emotional appeal into the levels of facts and insights. Let's say the patient asks what a veneer is. I'll answer by combining blue and red spectrum appeal, optimizing total appeal. Again, logic is in ***bold italics***, emotion in *regular italics*.

> ***"Mrs. Gowey, a veneer is man-made enamel that we bond to your teeth that strengthens and whitens them."***

> *"Just before I met you today, I saw Mabel, who had a situation just like yours. She hated the appearance of her teeth, was embarrassed to eat out, and last year we made her teeth solid again. They look great, and she loves it. You'll feel the same way, I'm sure."*

Notice figure 2. See how the intensity of appeal increases over time. The principle when using the Spectrum of Appeal is to escalate the appeal as you get further into the conversation.

Breakthrough and Hope

The highest levels of blue and red appeal are breakthrough and hope. These high levels of appeal are possible only after your listener has experienced the lower levels of appeal.

Facts pave the way to breakthroughs and insights open the heart to hope.

It's tough to give someone hope who doesn't know or like you, or has only a vague idea about what you do. The goal of the Spectrum of Appeal is to *build appeal in both spectrums* to the levels of breakthrough and hope. And once our listener has experienced the highest levels of appeal, red and blue, then we ask for action. Action makes sense following a breakthrough and feels good when accompanied by hope. (See figure 2.)

Spectrum Patterns

When mapping out the Spectrum of Appeal, patterns emerge. For example, figure 3 is a typical Spectrum of Appeal most dentists create during case presentation. I call this a "flat-liner," named after the EEG brain pattern that accompanies death. In this case it's death of persuasion, interest, and memorability. The "flat-liner" describes 95 percent of continuing education lectures. When a speaker "flat-lines" an audience, the listeners escape the dreariness by falling asleep. Have you ever been "flat-lined" at an association meeting or while in dental school? Join the club.

FIGURE 3: The "flat-line" blue spectrum: a typical dentist's case presentation

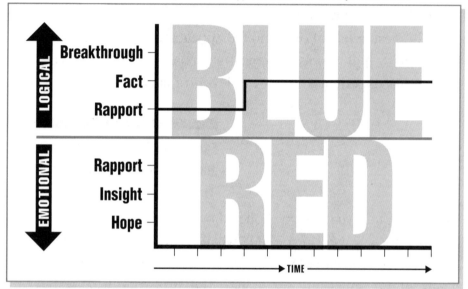

As audience members in dental continuing education we've all experienced great intellectuals who are rotten speakers. Their logic is so compelling, though, that we forgive the death-like delivery, chalk it up to eccentricity, and are happy to escape with a few "pearls." Patients are not as forgiving. If you have great intellect, are in private practice, *and* have a death-like delivery you'll have skinny kids.

I work with highly educated professionals in other industries such as engineering, financial services, and sales. These individuals share the fear that emotional appeal may compete with their credibility, perhaps diluting the impact of their message.

However, the appropriate amount of time spent in the emotional spectrum enhances credibility and strengthens the message because it makes the logic more digestible and interesting, and reduces "fanny fatigue." Remember: *You do not lose credibility by being interesting.* Logic is not ineffective in education or in case presentation, but it is incomplete.

> **Logic alone does not inspire people to act. If that were the case, no one would smoke or eat red meat and we'd all have fully funded pension plans.**

The "flat-line" red spectrum is as bad as the "flat-line" blue spectrum. (See figure 4.) This pattern is typical of people pleasers who so much want to be liked that they can't bring themselves to get to the point. In fact, they have no point. Too much emphasis in the emotional spectrum is called "baloney," named after the deli meat that's not good for you, and no one is sure what's in it. Too much "baloney" sends a mixed message: "I like my dentist to have a sense of humor, but I don't want Don Rickles rebuilding my mouth."

Diagnostic Spectral Patterns

Like ECG and EEG patterns that show what's going on inside the heart and brain respectively, spectral patterns demonstrate what's going on inside the heart and mind of the listener. Use these patterns to diagnose the style and impact of the speaker.

FIGURE 4: The "flat-line" red spectrum: too much "baloney."

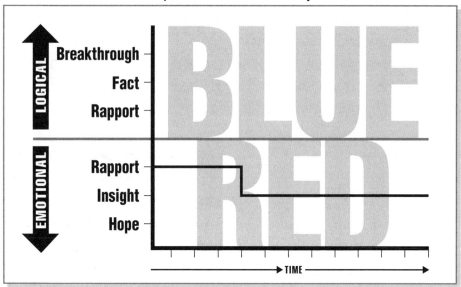

Figure 5 is the spectral pattern of one of the leading speakers in dentistry. Notice that the distribution of blue and red appeal is about 90/10, 90 percent blue, 10 percent red. This speaker's logic is compelling and he backs up his ideas and conclusions with considerable research and experience. This appeals to audiences of dentists who feed on new information. Notice, too, that from time to time this speaker will drop into the red spectrum. Usually this takes the form of a funny story illustrating his points.

He provides just enough red appeal to keep our attention and break up the abundance of blue appeal. He is a pleasure to listen to and he's very inspiring. His name is Dr. Gordon Christensen.

FIGURE 5: A sample of Dr. Gordon Christensen speaking 90% blue, 10% red.

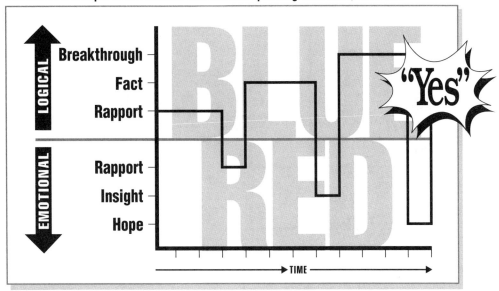

Figure 6 is a spectral pattern of another leading speaker. Notice his distribution of blue and red appeal is about 10/90, the opposite or Dr. Christensen's pattern. This speaker presents a concept, then beautifully and effortlessly illustrates his logic with wonderful stories. His stories are true accounts of dentists who have followed or not followed the concepts he's discussing. This speaker will go into the blue spectrum to make his point, and then justify and illustrate it in the red spectrum. This motivating speaker has enjoyed worldwide recognition for three decades, and his name is Dr. James Pride.

FIGURE 6: A sample of Dr. James Pride speaking 10% blue, 90% red.

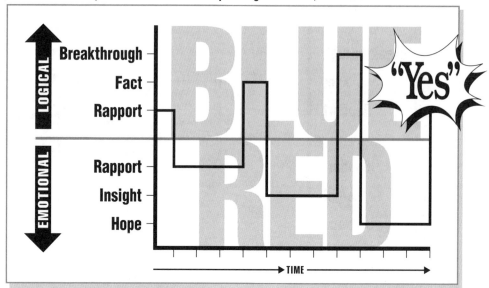

Illustrations: Think Red

In dentistry, where we have so much blue spectrum appeal, we need to search for red spectrum opposites to optimize appeal. Our blue spectrum language needs red spectrum illustration. Imagine you're in an airport and you walk up to a large magazine rack. What do you immediately notice? The pictures on the covers. These pictures illustrate what is in the magazine and are red spectrum tools used to trigger our interest. Journalists tell us that an article illustrated with photos, charts, and/or line drawings increases readership of the piece up to 800 percent! In fact, the captions under photos, which combine blue and red appeal, are the most frequently read element in a newspaper.

Our dental office language needs illustrations. I'm not talking about visual aids like study models and radiographs. We need to illustrate our blue spectrum language with red spectrum language, which provides broad appeal. That is exactly what Doctors Christensen and Pride have done. Both have built world-class organizations through their ability to appeal to those who support their organizations. The Spectrum of Appeal is the language of leadership and management.

> **All great leaders, in and outside of dentistry, have used broad appeal— blue and red—to inspire, motivate, and lead people toward meaningful growth.**

A Study in Contrast

It may seem that the spectrums used by Dr. Christensen and Dr. Pride are opposites. However, while their spectral patterns are opposite, the effect they have on the audience is identical; both speakers cause people to act, and both create enormous appeal for the same reasons. They combine opposites, blue and red, which create the contrast in their appeal that ignites and holds our interest. The element of contrast earns our interest and then holds our attention. The principle of creating contrast and interest by combining opposites is found in music, art, theater, literature, athletics, politics, entertainment, architecture, comedy, and in all types of relationships that include contrast: old and young, men and women, and so forth.

You create appeal when you
skillfully combine opposites.

Academic and Emotional Intelligence

In a book I highly recommend, *Working with Emotional Intelligence*, Daniel Goleman, Ph.D., offers a compelling discussion on the difference between academic and emotional intelligence. Academic intelligence is blue spectrum (see figure 7), which includes our IQ, training, and expertise. Academic intelligence is what qualified us to get into dental school and it determined our grades. Academic intelligence drives our intellectual ability, cognitive skills, technical know-how, and clinical treatment decisions.

FIGURE 7: Academic vs. emotional intelligence.

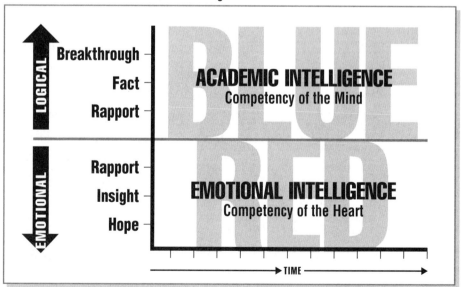

**Academic intelligence is the
competency of the mind.**

Emotional intelligence is red spectrum. It includes self-aware-ness, motivation, self-regulation, empathy, and social skills. Emotional intelligence allows us to build relationships with others, understand ourselves, have a drive to succeed, persuade others, and effectively use intuition.

**Emotional intelligence is the
competency of the heart.**

To succeed in dentistry, you need both academic and emotion-al intelligence. As Goleman says: *"Paradoxically, IQ has the least power in predicting success among the pool of people smart enough to handle the most cognitive demanding fields.*

In MBA programs or in careers like engineering, law, or med-icine, where professional selection focuses almost exclusively on intellectual abilities, emotional intelligence carries much more weight than IQ in determining who emerges as a leader."

To dentists and staff the greatest leverage and opportunity we have to build our careers involves learning to think, communi-cate, and act in the red spectrum. (See figure 8.) Dental school focuses on academic intelligence. Because we are rewarded and advanced in school based on academic intelligence, our emo-tional intelligence can atrophy in the process. But remember the adage, "Use it or lose it." It applies to emotional intelligence, too.

FIGURE 8: The greatest opportunities we have to build our dental careers exist in the emotional (red) spectrum.

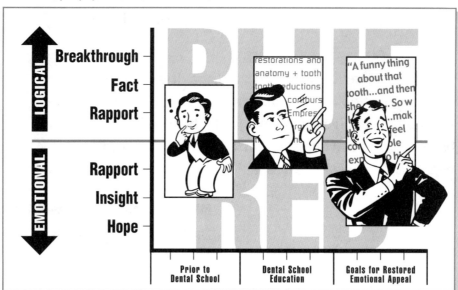

Goleman explains that emotional intelligence does not mean just being nice to people. Emotional intelligence is the way to leverage our knowledge and skills; it's another way of being smart. Lack of emotional intelligence makes smart people look stupid.

Academic and Emotional Memory

Has this ever happened to you? You're driving down the street; you flip on the radio and hear an old song you used to listen to years ago when you were in loooooove. From deep inside, emotion and fond memories pour out like a river. Did you have to struggle to recall those memories or did they just leap out on their own? What you've just experienced is emotional memory.

(See figure 9.) It is hard to forget how we feel, and in fact, it's automatic, even when you don't want to remember your feelings about bad childhood experiences or brushes with death.

Emotional memory contrasts with cognitive memory, which involves recalling facts, figures, and data. This is the memory we use to get through school and jump through the hoops related to licensure and certifications. Cognitive memory is what we are rewarded for in the social, political, and academic structure of dentistry.

Have you ever forgotten someone's name, your ATM code, and the combination to the lock of your health club locker? Of course—memory lapses of this type are so common we think of them as routine. But have you ever forgotten how you feel about any person, place, or thing? That would be rare in human experience.

FIGURE 9: Academic vs. emotional memory.

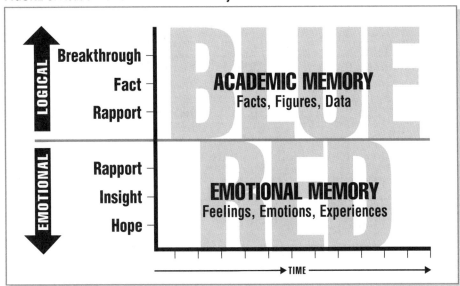

It requires no effort to access emotional memory and it endures for a lifetime. *When emotion is attached to an experience, it anchors the memory.*

What do you want patients to remember about you? Most of my dentist clients spend their time and effort with patients reciting treatment recommendations, information, and patient education. Of course we'd like patients to remember our treatment recommendations and information, but what they actually remember is if they liked you and your staff and how they feel about the process. Patients will forget what you said to them, but they'll remember whether they liked you or not. Patients remember more what they feel than what they hear.

Academic and Emotional Speed

Our capacity to cognitively process information—academic speed—is fast. (See figure 10.) According to estimates we can think at several hundred words per minute. Prove this to yourself. Visualize (a cognitive process) the following items as fast as you can read them: hill, house, barn, dog, cat, snake, cloud, raisin, and mother. No problem I'm sure. Now try to experience the following emotions: hate, love, fear, confidence, loneliness, and bravery. You notice it takes much longer to identify your feelings.

Identifying our feelings takes time. Complete care patients may not fully understand how they feel about you until well after they hear your treatment recommendations. Give them time. Don't push for treatment acceptance decisions too fast. Most people need time to process the information and impressions. I am *against* "going for the close" at the first or second

FIGURE 10: We operate at mental speed, but our patients operate at emotional speed.

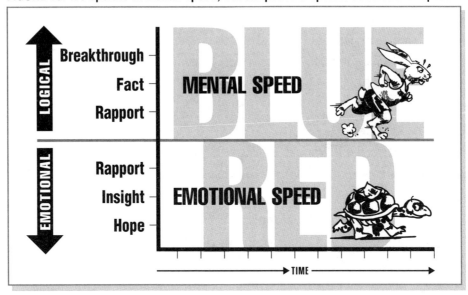

What are patients most likely to remember after they leave your office, your technical explanations or how they felt about the experience? In the dental office, dentists and staff think, act, and speak at mental speed. But complete care patients operate at emotional speed.

appointments. Slick closes that offer a list of alternative choices push people into decisions they may not be ready to make. A quick decision makes little difference at the tooth dentistry level; but before I start a major rehabilitation, I want my patients to feel good about their choices, and those choices take time.

Designing Brochures

The Spectrum of Appeal applies to printed material as well. Design your brochures and promotional materials using a 20/80 ratio, 20 percent logic, and 80 percent emotion. Other than consent and financial documents, the 20/80 ratio is good for patient-targeted literature and promotional materials. While your target patients are processing their decision to accept your care, your 20/80 printed material will support them and reinforce the attitude of your office.

The 20/80 ratio is true for everything patients see on the walls of your office. What would have greater appeal to a patient: a close-up technical photograph with lips retracted showing a before-and-after cosmetic result, or a full-face photograph of a happy patient with a great letter of appreciation? And how about that poster that shows the progression of periodontal disease from a healthy mouth to advanced periodontitis, including close-up photographs of very nasty teeth and gums. How much appeal does this have? It's time to take down all the photographs and illustrations that showcase disease. I'm very glad some dentists I know don't practice urology!

The Language of Leadership and Management

Let's use the Spectrum of Appeal to map the patterns of management and leadership. Figure 11 shows a management pattern. This pattern shows an instructing, mentoring language, with the most emphasis on the blue spectrum: facts, how to, when, where, how many, and so forth. The blue/red ratio is about 80/20.

This 80/20 pattern is also the pattern of traditional sales techniques. Many of the techniques of sales—prospecting, getting the appointment, presenting benefits and features, overcoming objections, closing—are blue spectrum. Spectra of management and traditional sales are quite similar.

FIGURE 11: Management pattern of 80% blue, 20% red.

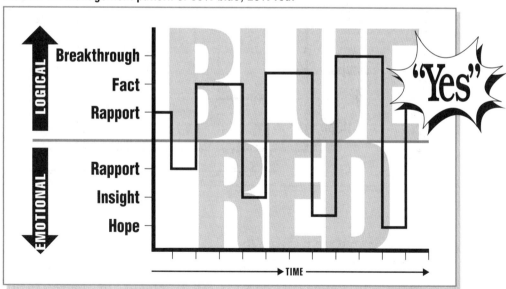

Figure 12 is a leadership pattern. This pattern shows a coaching, illustrative, intuitive pattern with most of the emphasis on the red spectrum—reasons, encouragement, character, vision. The blue-red ratio is about 20/80. Think back, who made the biggest difference in your life? Chances are excellent that he or she had a leadership pattern. The leadership pattern supports the management pattern. When you stimulate the appropriate emotion, when you show someone the possibility for hope, growth occurs.

FIGURE 12: Leadership pattern 20% blue, 80% red.

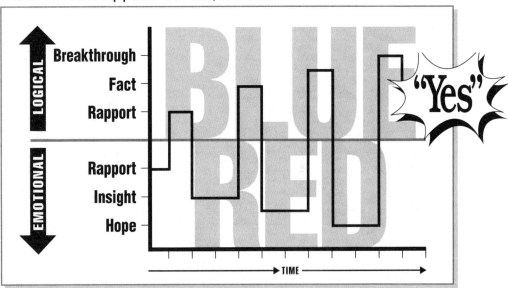

Case Acceptance Patterns

When an expert is trying to influence, to appeal to another expert, the language pattern is 80/20. This is the management/ sales pattern. (See figure 13.) If I am a dental equipment dealer (an expert) and am trying to sell you (also an expert) a digital

x-ray unit, I will try to influence you using what is most familiar to you, the blue spectrum. You and I speak the same language: logic. Although great salespeople can leverage their
logical appeal with emotional appeal, the bulk of the dialogue
in this situation falls into the blue spectrum: benefits, features,
costs, delivery, maintenance, warranties. Another word for blue
spectrum dialogue is jargon. Experts and managers speak jargon
to each other because they understand its meaning.

**When an expert is trying to influence
a novice, the expert must speak the
same language as the novice.**

FIGURE 13: Experts speaking to experts 80% blue, 20% red.

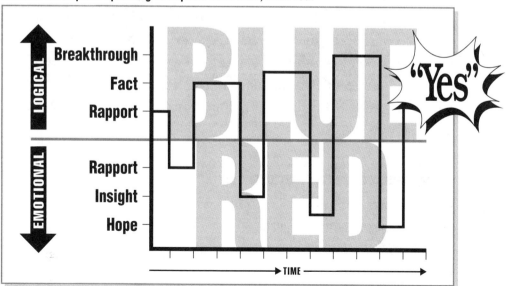

FIGURE 14: Experts speaking to novices 20% blue, 80% red.

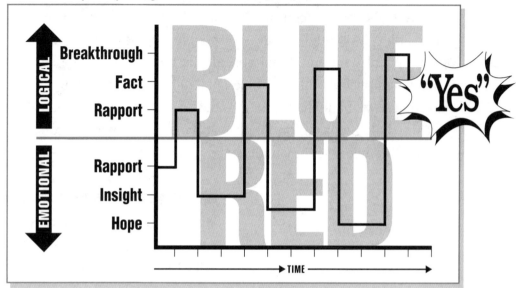

Take a look at figure 14. The language pattern here is 20/80, the leadership pattern. For example, if you're a real-estate salesperson and you're dealing with first-time buyers, you'll do well if you focus your language on areas most familiar to your buyers: neighborhood, schools, shopping, churches. The smart real-estate salesperson doesn't use words like easements, footings, deeds-of-trust, or eminent domain. Jargon doesn't work on novices.

With the novice, the expert minimizes blue spectrum language because it has little meaning, hence little appeal.

Case acceptance is an expert-to-novice dialogue (See figure 14.) Compare the case acceptance pattern to the leadership pattern in figure 12. You'll find they are identical, which offers a profound insight into the case acceptance process.

Structurally, case acceptance for complete dentistry is the leadership pattern.

Do sales and leadership have different meanings to you? Look at figure 15. Traditional selling is a blue spectrum skill. Traditional sales skills include asking questions to evaluate the prospect's needs, uncovering buyer motivators and "hot buttons," presenting features and benefits, overcoming objections, asking for the order, asking for referrals.

FIGURE 15: Case acceptance is a blend of selling and leadership.

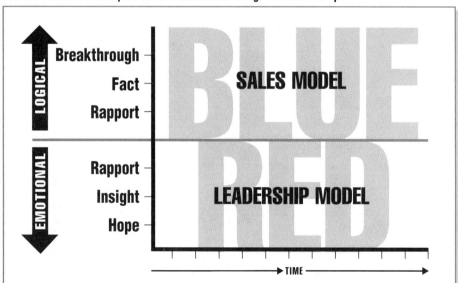

Leadership is a red spectrum skill. Leaders know their own strengths and weaknesses, show confidence and self-control, are motivating, are aware of others feelings, and are adept at influencing others. Case acceptance is a blend of selling and leadership, with greater emphasis on leadership.

Are you more comfortable selling something or leading someone? Most dentists are far more comfortable leading than they are selling, but structurally the two skills are similar. The difference is in the attitude of the expert. If you feel better when leading as opposed to selling, then lead your patients into case acceptance, rather than attempting to sell them into it.

When your attitude is that of a leader, the fear of sounding like a salesperson disappears.

Questions and Objections

Let's put typical blue spectrum questions and objections on the Spectrum of Appeal. (See figure 16.) *"What is the cap made of?"* *"How do you do it?"* *"How will you fix my tooth?"* *"What makes my tooth hurt?"* These are common blue spectrum questions or comments. They seek information.

Let's put typical red spectrum questions/comments on the Spectrum of Appeal. *"Why is it so expensive?"* *"I'm afraid it will hurt,"* *"I'm disappointed my insurance won't pay,"* *"Do I really need this much dentistry?"* *"How much longer will it take?"*

Compare the blue and red spectrum questions/comments. Which spectrum represents the questions/comments that make or break case acceptance? Red, of course. But where do we spend most of our time explaining things and where are we the most comfortable? Blue, of course.

> In terms of case acceptance for complete dentistry, we spend most of our time and energy in areas that matter least.

Be aware that some questions may sound like blue spectrum information-seeking questions, but may be red spectrum questions based on emotions, such as fear or loss of control. For example, *"How much does it cost?"* sounds like a request for facts, in this case the cost of the dentistry itself, or on the surface, blue spectrum information. But for most patients the red spectrum question *"Can I afford it?"* lurks in the back-

FIGURE 16: Objections and questions.

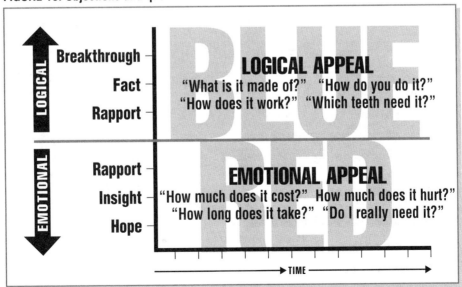

ground. The concept of affordability, literally the ability to buy, relates to safety, which is a red spectrum issue for most people.

Stay in the patient's spectrum. The key to answering questions and comments using the Spectrum of Appeal is to give your answer in the same spectrum as the question. If you hear a blue spectrum question, *"When is my appointment?"* reply in the blue spectrum: *"Your appointment is tomorrow."* If you hear a red spectrum question or remark: *"I'm afraid it will it hurt,"* reply in the red spectrum: *"It's normal to feel afraid, and many of my patients are afraid. We make sure everyone is comfortable and safe in our office. We'll do the same for you."* Answer questions and objections in the spectrum in which they originated. Don't make the patient come to you, you go to the patient. If your answer doesn't work, change the spectrum.

For example, your patient asks, *"How long will my care take?"* You interpret this as a blue spectrum question and respond in the blue spectrum, *"Your care will take one year to complete."* He rejects your answer and tells you that his job won't allow him to take the time. Instead of staying in the blue spectrum and proceeding to recite reasons and facts why quality care takes time, change your spectrum to red. *"Adam, I've treated many businessmen like you and I'm great about respecting your work schedules and commitments. I recently finished a CEO just like you, and he missed very little work. I will do the same for you."*

**If your answer doesn't work,
change your spectrum.**

Most dentists have a default spectrum, one that they're most comfortable with. Usually it's blue. When confronted with objections, questions, or stress, dentists usually slip into the default blue spectrum because it's easy.

Think about all the objections you've heard. In which spectrum do most fall? Red. Most objections that are case acceptance busters are in the red spectrum. *To enjoy case acceptance of complete dentistry, a dentist and staff must learn red spectrum skills.*

Overcoming Objections

The phrase "overcoming objections" comes to us from the world of sales. The inference we can draw is that I, as the salesperson, will use my logic and wit to change your mind about your resistance to purchase what I'm selling. For example, if my buyer has issues related to costs, I'll give him facts, data, proof that the purchase is worth it, is a good investment, and so forth. I may use emotion and push a few hot buttons or remind the buyer of his motivators.

In dentistry, I challenge the concept of overcoming objections, specifically, the word "overcoming." To overcome something connotes a contest or breaking a barrier, in this case, a contest between the dentist and patient. It's almost as if patients are wrong in stating their objections, and it's our job as dentists to correct them. Considering that most objections are red spectrum, that is, emotional objections, we breed animosity if we tell our patients that how they feel is wrong.

The fastest way to make others mad is to tell them they're wrong about how they feel.

Instead of "overcoming" the objection, acknowledge it. Don't make patients wrong because they are afraid, or believe the care is too expensive, or are disappointed by the lack of insurance coverage. Acknowledge their emotions and give them the space to be right. Your job as the professional is to move to their emotional place and then offer an insight that may help them see another way of looking at the situation.

Answering Questions and Acknowledging Objections

No rigid pattern for patient dialogues exists, so do not spend time looking for one right answer. The secret to creating the most appeal is to recognize where the patient is and comfortably move between spectrums. Here's a good template to follow (see figure 17), which illustrates three basic ways to respond: direct, defer, or illustrate.

The direct answer occupies the blue spectrum. It is the best response to a direct question. For example, you're asked, *"How much will my insurance pay?"* A direct answer would be: *"Your insurance limitation is 1,200 dollars per year. In your case, insurance will pay 50 percent of the total fee for this crown."* Blue spectrum question, direct blue spectrum response.

However, there are times when a direct answer will take your dialogue down a path you don't want to travel. Deferring the answer might be a better strategy. For example, you're asked,

"How much will my insurance pay?" A deferral sounds like this: *"I'll know better how much your insurance will pay after I've planned your care."* Deferring this question will give you more opportunity to build rapport with this patient, so when you do answer this question directly, there's a greater chance the patient will take your advice over the insurance company's. A deferral occupies a neutral spectrum, with no commitment to blue or red.

FIGURE 17: Acknowledging questions and objections—three types of responses.

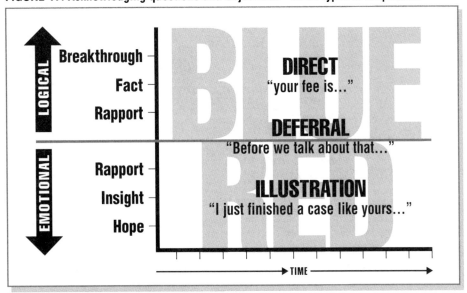

Answering a question with a question is a form of deferral. For example, you're asked about insurance. A deferral in the form of question may sound like: *"Is insurance coverage an important concern for you?"* Your answer to your patient's question now guides you to your best response, either a direct answer or an illustration.

The third way to answer a question is to use an illustration, a story, metaphor, simile, humor, comparison, or testimony. The illustration answer is a red spectrum response. I recommend using an illustration whenever it's clear that you have a red spectrum question. For example, your patient says: *"I am so disappointed that my insurance isn't going to pay for my dentistry. I've worked all these years paying for it and you'd think it would be worth something."*

You must realize that there is no graceful and effective way to answer this objection directly or with a deferral, and the situation would likely become worse. Instead, use an illustration: *"Joe, I have a patient in this practice that was just as disappointed as you in his insurance and he put off his dentistry. On the way to the airport, a cap on his front tooth came off. We fixed it for him and he caught the later flight. His insurance didn't help him much, but we did. We'll do the same for you."* The illustration does not provide blue spectrum information. Rather it shows how another patient was frustrated but overcame the frustration and now is happy with the result.

Effectively use the three ways to answer a question by being aware of where the patient is and where you are in the Spectrum of Appeal. And if your answer doesn't work, change spectrums. Let's say you have a new patient and from what your staff tells you, she is a rehabilitative patient. You've done an initial examination and she has advanced dental disease in all areas of her mouth. You'd like the opportunity to study her case and create a treatment plan for her. However, patients sometimes act in normal yet unacceptable ways (from your viewpoint), and this patient asks point-blank how much you will charge her to fix her teeth. Here's a sample dialogue using all three ways of answering the same question: *"How much will it cost to fix my teeth?"*

Using deferral, I answer: *"I'll know better after I study your case, Mrs. Breiding. I suggest I study your case when you're not here, and when you return, I'll know your case by heart."*

"Yeah, I know," she says, *"but you've done cases like mine before, give me a ballpark estimate."* She's pushing for an answer.

Using a direct answer, I say: *"A case like yours will cost 12,000 dollars and will take about a year to complete. Does that fit within your budget?"*

"I had no idea dentistry could cost that much. What makes it so expensive?" she asks.

Using illustration, I say: *"Many patients tell me the same thing. You remind me of Sally. We finished her case three years ago. She suffered with bad teeth all her life. It was after she saw what wearing dentures did to her husband that she started her care with us. Yes, it's expensive, but Sally considered losing her teeth more expensive. We stayed within Sally's budget and we'll do the same for you."*

When deferring an answer, be prepared for an objection to the deferral. If you hear one, give a direct answer or an illustration.

Don't be like a deer caught in the headlights with your default blue spectrum direct responses. These often work to make patients appear wrong and, therefore, a contest starts. I'm not saying that blue spectrum responses are wrong. But as I've said before, they're incomplete with respect to using the entire range of the Spectrum of Appeal.

Case Presentation Patterns

Typical case presentations spectral patterns appear in figure 18. This is an 80/20 pattern: 80 percent logic, 20 percent emotion. The dentist begins the presentation in the blue spectrum by reciting the findings and diagnosis. Sometime soon the patient asks a question, makes a comment, or raises an objection. Most of the time these questions/comments/objections fall in the red spectrum. Most dentists I work with will respond to red spectrum issues in the blue spectrum and give more facts and proof. The presentation continues until the next questions/comments/objections, at which point the dentist escalates the logic, providing even stronger evidence that supports treatment recommendations. Patients get the facts, but they don't experience emotional appeal. Why should it surprise us that patients say no?

When speaking with patients, you must minimize blue spectrum language because it has little meaning, hence little appeal.

Michael Sunich, Ed.d., a psychologist practicing in Charlotte, North Carolina, proposes the following illustration. (See figure 19.) As the dentist talks about the problems in the patient's mouth, the patient feels concern. Too often instead of acknowledging and supporting the concern, the dentist presses on and outlines the solutions, which can bring on frustration from the patient because he doesn't feel heard. Now the dentist experiences the consequences of not treating the emotional

FIGURE 18: An unsuccessful pattern of case acceptance.

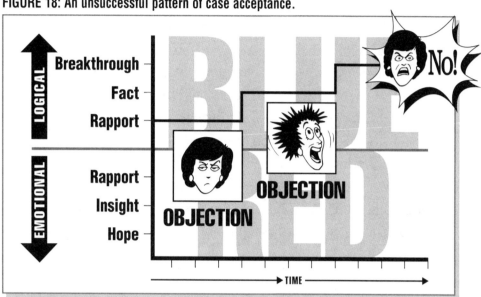

FIGURE 19: Escalating negative emotional appeal.

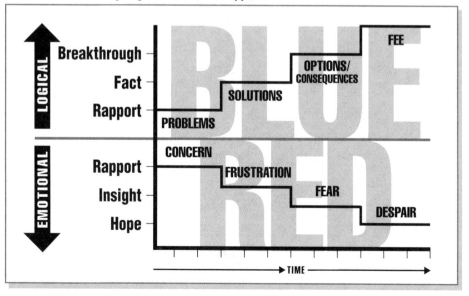

"condition," which can bring on fear. And just when the patient is feeling worse, at the worst possible point in the patient's level of appeal, the dentist quotes the fee. Because the patient has accumulated unacknowledged negative feelings, the fee can represent an insurmountable emotional wall; instead of experiencing hope, the patient feels despair.

So, do you want your complete care patients to experience fear and frustration when they hear your fee? What will patients remember best, your care, skill, and judgment, or the despair they felt when they heard the fee? What do you think they'll tell their friends about their trip to the dentist?

Figure 20 illustrates a more successful spectral pattern of case presentations. This is a 20/80 pattern, 20 percent logic, 80 percent emotion. Again, the dentist begins the presentation in the blue spectrum by reciting the findings and diagnosis. The patient soon asks a question, makes a comment, or states an objection. Now, instead of offering more facts to overcome the objection, the dentist shifts to the red spectrum and offers insight (understanding) to the facts presented. This is done through the use of empathy, a story, comparison, a metaphor, and so on.

After patients have had adequate time to process the insight, the dentist continues with the presentation, making additional recommendations for care. Soon another question/comment/objection is forthcoming (usually red spectrum) and as before, the dentist shifts to the red spectrum, and offers insights/understanding into the emotions the patient feels at this point in the process. Only after patients experience the emotions of insight and understanding are they able to sense that there is hope for them. Insights lead to hope, but facts do not. When patients experience hope, they may have a breakthrough and see that you are the answer to their dental problems.

Facts are useless unless the patient experiences insights into them. A lot of facts do not equate to a lot of understanding and appeal.

Hope and breakthroughs are faithful companions. When patients experience hope, they'll often have the breakthrough and see the way to dental health, specifically, through *your care*. Patients who see the way to dental health have hope, which then supports and drives their decision to accept care.

When presenting fees, the best possible level of emotional appeal for the patient is hope.

Study the patterns in this chapter and notice how most of what we do in case presentation is in the blue spectrum. Nearly every dentist I work with structures case acceptance based on an 80/20 structure. They predominately use blue spectrum activities, which is a sales model, and focus on quality, patient education, a show-and-tell technical approach to communication, and dealing with the limitations of dental insurance. These same dentists all ask me to help them with the same issues: They want to do more dentistry on fewer patients, reduce their stress, and make more money. In every case where dentists learn a 20/80 red spectrum approach, they see an increase in complete care, low-volume, and low-stress dentistry.

A very clear relationship exists between 80/20 blue spectrum case-acceptance patterns and low-fee, high-volume, stressful tooth dentistry.

FIGURE 20: A successful pattern of case acceptance.

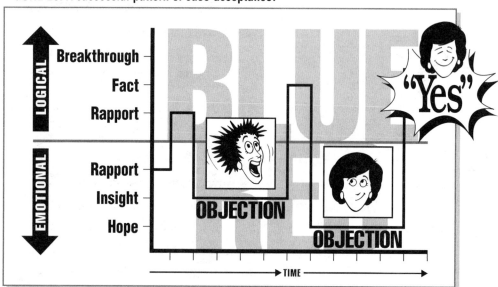

As I've said, blue spectrum 80/20 case-acceptance patterns are not wrong, but they are incomplete. In our country we enjoy the highest standard of care in the world. Blue spectrum case-acceptance techniques are responsible for the overwhelming majority of the dentistry done in our country. However, when I look at the dentists who are consistently doing the high-fee complete care cases, I always see strong 20/80 red spectrum patterns in the dentist, the staff, or both.

Beyond "Yes"

Whether you use an 80/20 or 20/80 style, the goal is the same. You want your patients to say yes to your strategy for complete care. (See figure 21.) We can argue that if you can get to yes by either style, what difference does it make? The difference is apparent in what happens after the coveted "yes." The only thing 80/20 and 20/80 have in common is that you can get a positive response from either method. But that's where the similarity ends.

Beyond "yes," the 20/80 style brings you and your team a better relationship with the patient. This relationship enhances all of the positive responses occurring during and after treatment is complete. (See figure 22.) The 20/80 style helps you with:

1. **Commitment:** Patients are motivated to follow through with treatment or return if they postpone treatment.
2. **Clinical management:** Reduces stress and creates a more therapeutic atmosphere.
3. **Collections:** People who like you, pay you.
4. **Insurance:** Patients adopt your opinion, not the insurance company's.

FIGURE 21: The goal is to get patients to "Yes."

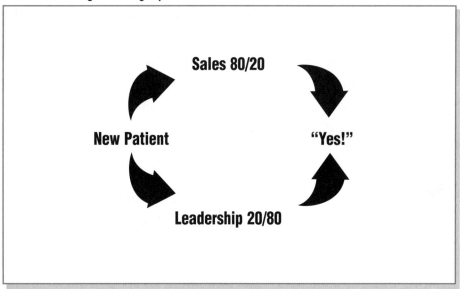

FIGURE 22: Beyond "Yes"

	80/20	20/80
Relationship		✔
Commitment		✔
Clinical Mgt.		✔
Collections		✔
Insurance		✔
Recall		✔
Referral		✔
Mgt. of failures		✔
Medical/Legal		✔
Profitability		✔

5. **Recall:** Patients are willing to follow your instructions.
6. **Referral:** People who like you tell their friends about you.
7. **Management of failures:** Re-treatment issues are less stressful.
8. **Medical/legal:** Patients who like you are less likely to sue you.
9. **Profitability:** You'll make more money and experience less stress when treating cooperative complete care patients.

The Lesson

The lesson is simple. If you want to do more comprehensive complete care cases, learn red spectrum skills. But it's human nature to resist change, and I've had clients ask if I could help them sell bigger cases without using that "warm, fuzzy red spectrum stuff." The answer is yes, but to do it you have to create a marketing machine that produces a parade of new patients for your practice. Then once they're in your chair, use your 80/20 blue spectrum, drive-by style, show-and-tell case presentation pattern, and sell one out of fifty complete care cases. When they seek my services, most of my clients are running their practices that way, and now they want to learn a new approach.

When clients want to bypass the "warm fuzzy" approach, I just tell them that when they start marketing, they'll hear no more often, make even less money, and have much more stress. So, if you want to practice complete care dentistry and live to tell about it, you'll need to learn red spectrum skills. If you are reading this book because you want to get to the "next level," then you've got to stop trying to sell things to people and start building relationships.

CHAPTER 5

Sounds Like You KNOW WHAT You're TALKING About

Tools of Expression

Are dentists who sound like they know what they're talking about more successful than those who don't? Does a bear floss in the woods? No communication or sales technique will sell complete dentistry every time. Not everyone will say yes to what you offer, but if you're memorable and persuasive, your message won't be forgotten.

In the previous chapter I talked about red spectrum language tools. The four major red spectrum language tools include **attitude, connection, disclosure, and visual language**. Blend these tools into the logic of your presentation and you'll go a long way in becoming more interesting, memorable, and persuasive.

It Starts with Attitude

Attitude is best characterized as the emotion behind your words. When we're clear about how we feel about a topic, our tone of voice, posture, breathing, and gestures come to life.

The big giveaway that reveals your attitude is your tone of voice.

Your tone of voice accounts for up to *35 percent* of the impact on your listeners. Contrast that with the fact that only 10 percent of your impact comes from the meaning of the words you use, even less if you use jargon. You usually can't hide the emotion in your voice, whether it's anger, confusion, fear, joy, or delight. Occasionally my wife Carolyn will snap, "Don't use that tone of voice with me!" Her issue is not so much the tone of my voice, but rather my attitude, or the emotion she senses is behind the words. Tone of voice signals how we feel, which is another way of describing our attitude at that time.

When speaking on the telephone, tone of voice is even more influential. It's estimated that our tone of voice accounts for up to 85 percent of our impact during telephone conversations.

Scripted Responses

A major objection I have to dentists and staff who use a script or pat answers in response to patients' questions or objections is that we lose our personal attitude. The more we focus on saying the right words, the less animated our voices become. Patients can sense when you slip into a scripted response because of your tone of voice.

Rigid scripted responses are not effective or desirable under any circumstances. Certainly, these scripted structures such as critical dialogues help us learn verbal skills. But as soon as you learn the structure of the response, stop thinking about saying the right words and allow your feelings to come through.

Body Language

A speaker's body is the most powerful visual aid he or she has. When we're in touch with the emotions, the passion behind our words, then the body follows. Movement is language. Up to 60 percent of our impact on listeners is visual and is communicated through movement, body language, facial expression, and posture. Our passion inspires our movement. If a speaker isn't moving it's hard to imagine that she has strong beliefs about the topic. If the speaker does not have passion about the topic, why should the listeners be passionate about it?

If you're not passionate about great dentistry, don't expect your patients to be excited either.

I've read a lot about body language. Most of what I've read and heard sounds like this: "If you want to convince someone of something, then sit like this." "If you want to build rapport, then stand like that…"

The problem I have with consciously using the body to influence others is that it can be stiff and reek of learned and practiced technique, which comes across as lifeless as a rehearsed monologue. Let your passion move you naturally and your listeners will experience your passion and be moved into action.

Get Real

It's important to keep in mind that attitude, which in essence means learning to get in touch with the emotion behind your words, does not mean that you're wildly enthusiastic and unrealistically upbeat each time you speak. Attitude will change from time to time. There are times when your attitude may be mellow, humorous, supportive, and so on. Attitude must change based on circumstances or you lose your credibility and the interest of your listeners. Again: *No one has ever lost credibility by being interesting.*

Since 1995 I've taught a two-day workshop called "Speaking of Dentistry" in which I coach speakers on being more memorable and persuasive. I often see speakers who are reluctant to demonstrate how they feel about their topic; in other words, they resist red spectrum patterns. These speakers believe that the logic of their presentation is sufficient to persuade audiences. However, speakers boost their persuasiveness, credibility, and likability by 100 percent once they give themselves permission to demonstrate and give voice their attitude.

To sell complete care dentistry, you must demonstrate your attitude during the process of getting to know new patients. When your attitude is obvious through your movement and tone of voice, patients feel as if they have gotten through to you and you're interested in them. Your attitude, a red spectrum skill, demonstrates that interest.

Before patients become interested and committed, you must first demonstrate significant interest in them.

Making a Connection

A patient feels connected when you give him or her your full attention, and invariably makes the patient feel important. Connection is a powerful foundation on which to build rapport, and for that reason, connection is a powerful red spectrum tool. Like attitude, if you want your patients' full attention, you must first give them your full attention, which you demonstrate through eye connection, voice quality, proximity, and humor.

Making an Eye Connection

You've no doubt heard about the importance of eye contact. Eye connection takes eye contact to a higher level. By that I mean that eye connection means looking into your patient's eyes as you've looked into a child's eyes to earn his attention. When you're speaking to children about something important, do you look away or make fleeting eye contact? Not likely! You look into a child's eyes until you see the "lights go on." You can tell if the child understands and trusts you, and you sense likes, dislikes, and fears by the look in his or her eyes. It isn't any different with most adults.

Connecting gives your patient the opportunity to look into your eyes. Patients can tell a lot about you by the look in your eye. They can tell if you're distracted, nervous, tired, or angry. Let them see that you're accepting, open, interested, kind, humorous, and gentle. Is it important to give patients the opportunity to "read" your eyes? If you want to sell complete dentistry, it certainly is.

Most dentists don't connect. Instead, they make brief eye contact and then look away and speak as if they were reading from a script. When I do case acceptance consulting for complete dentistry in-office, I've discovered that dentists do the same thing with their patients, only worse.

Most dentists talk to their patients while simultaneously looking at their records, a radiograph, a study model, or even while staring off into space. Staff members do the same. The most consistent eye contact with the patient occurs when the dentists say hello and goodbye.

Stress is a sure way to disconnect us. John Gray, Ph.D., author of *Men Are from Mars, Women Are from Venus*, says: "What gets in between men and relationships is stress." When I coach dentists in communication skills, I've noticed male dentists are more prone to disconnect during a conversation. Stress also destroys our tone of voice. That said, stress is part of dentistry and we can only seek ways to cope with it and minimize it as much as possible. For example, in the section on case acceptance structure I'll discuss why blocking examination and consultation appointments together helps reduce the stress.

Don't confuse connection with eye contact. Connection is giving someone your full attention, and eye contact is part of that process. We've all met people, usually salespeople, who make eye contact, but you know something is lacking. They are not making a true connection with you because they aren't giving you their full attention. They aren't actually listening to you, because they're thinking of their next response. In all likelihood, these salespeople are thinking about their lists of benefits and features and considering ways to coax you to overcome your objections. These are people who want you to get to the point so they can make theirs. Eye contact by itself is a sales technique, but does not guarantee a connection. Connection is emotional appeal.

> **Connection is the experience a person has when you give that person your full attention.**

High-Tech, Low Connection

One of the disadvantages of the high-tech world of the modern dental office is that it can disconnect patients and doctors. Most technology is a blue spectrum tool. Of course, I am not against having the best technology in your office, but I am against relying on it to sell complete dentistry. Human contact can easily be lost when we rely on intraoral images, CD-based patient education, and visual aids.

In early 1998 I was doing in-office case acceptance coaching for a client in Florida. During this visit, I played the role of a new patient. As we went through the new patient procedure, the assistant seated me in the patient's chair in the operatory and plugged in a twelve-minute videotape. The video explained periodontal disease, the periodontal examination, and the value of the complete examination. It was the longest twelve minutes of my life. Then the doctor came in and asked me if I had any questions about the tape!

Yes, the videotape was efficient. It used technology instead of human effort to explain things. But was it effective? Did I have any greater sense about a relationship with the dentist? Did I connect with the dentist or staff? No indeed. We *want* technology to be the answer to case acceptance. It's the easy solution.

Just think, buy a bunch of high-tech stuff and the patients will roll over and say yes! This is the "If you buy it, they will come" philosophy of case acceptance.

―――――――――――

Technology has never been the answer to case acceptance for complete care.

Back in the 1970s the high-tech "must-haves" were fully adjustable articulators and phase contrast microscopes. Did they sell complete cases? Would you like to buy some used articulators or microscopes? The '80s and '90s ushered in a plethora of high-tech items, and most dentists have bought their fair share. Technology has made dentistry and administrating dental practices technically easier, but has technology made complete care dentistry easier to sell? Most dentists, especially the ones who have bought a lot of high-tech items, would say no.

People cannot connect with a picture or a model. Intraoral pictures are great for showing a split tooth, thick calculus, and selling low-fee tooth dentistry. Low-fee tooth dentistry is a commodity in dentistry. I've already explained the difference between selling complete and tooth dentistry. When you sell tooth care you're selling the commodity—the crown, the veneer, the root canal. With complete dentistry, you're selling you and your capacity to build and maintain solid relationships with your patients. Technology can get in the way of building relationships.

During one of my programs a specialist said: "If I want a person to feel important, I do a very thorough examination. If they've never had a really thorough examination, they'll feel important when we're done."

I agree that clinical thoroughness makes patients feel good. But in terms of building rapport, the thoroughness of an examination, which is blue spectrum material, is chicken feed compared to your ability to connect, which is obvious red spectrum activity.

Knowing When to Connect

There are two times when you absolutely must connect with a patient. You must connect when you're quoting the fee and delivering bad news because both are red spectrum events for your patient. During these conversations you must thoroughly demonstrate your confidence, believability, and ethics. Ironically, these are the most common times when my clients will disconnect and look at the patient's record or off into space.

Remember what I said in chapter 4: *Go to the spectrum your patient is in.* In general, it is stressful to discuss money and bad news, so disconnecting may *seem* normal during these conversations, but it is still unacceptable. Understand that I'm not advocating a rigid stare. It's natural to briefly look away momentarily while searching for your words. Just don't look away for too long and when you do, smile and stay connected.

Voice Quality

The quality of your voice can help connect you to your patient. The pace, or rhythm, of your voice is an important component of voice quality. The pace of your voice is actually the silence between the thoughts, the pauses. Patients need time to think while we're talking. If you run all your words together, patients can't keep up. Patients need time to identify how they feel about what you're saying, which goes back to the concept of emotional vs. mental speed. Just as sentences are punctuated with commas, spaces, hyphens, periods, and paragraph indents, so too, must our spoken language be punctuated with pauses to let the message sink in and to gain insight from your facts.

Don't confuse pace with rate. *Rate is how fast you speak; pace is the pause between thoughts.* Your speaking rate is rarely too fast if you allow sufficient pauses between ideas. The sexes tend to react differently to stress and this is reflected in speech. Stress tends to disconnect male dentists and they narrow their focus to blue spectrum issues. Female dentists under stress tend to increase their rate (words per minute) of speech, and decrease the pace (pause between thoughts). To generalize, stress makes men talk less and women talk more. Both responses can disconnect you from patients.

Your Sense of Humor

Do you believe it is important to use humor in the dental office? If you want to sell complete-care cases it is extremely important because humor opens people up. Humor can be the ultimate red spectrum skill. It makes you seem human, full of life, and a "regular" person. Humor distances you from the stereotype of the "dull dentist."

In some dental office situations humor is the only answer. In 1994 my associate referred a wonderful woman from his church to my practice. She was as big as a house, her hair was blue, and she had an abscess half the size of a hard-boiled egg. She was scared to death and nothing was going to ease her fear.

As I approached her I was going to say, "Open up, I need to take a look." But I was thinking, "Open up, I need to take a peek." Instead, I said, "Open up, I need to take a leak!" Lisa, my assistant, fell off her chair and the three of us had a great laugh. Before the patient knew it, she had been numbed for the procedure and was comfortable. Humor is a mandatory skill in dentistry. Its ability to connect people is unmatched.

> **The next time you're tempted to take another course on technical dentistry, stop yourself and consider a course on humor, stand-up comedy, or humorous theatrical technique.**

Proximity

Have you ever been to a party and someone comes up to you and stands just a little too close? What do you do? You back away. In our culture the space, or "zone of comfort," between two men is a little more than an arm's distance; the comfort zone is a bit less than an arm's distance between a man and woman, and the distance closes still more for two women. If you doubt this is true, you need only look around in public spaces and you will see these three basic "comfort zones" that dictate our proximity to each other.

In the dental office, we get closer than what people would normally tolerate, and patients usually do not have the option of backing away. Because we work in close proximity, our ability to connect is crucially important. If you have connected well by using eye contact, voice, and humor, then the closer you get to the patient, the more favorable effect you have. If you have not connected well with your patient, the closer you get the more anxious he or she feels. Since we must be close to patients to perform our job, connections become critical.

When you learn how to connect with people, your proximity becomes therapeutic.

Self-disclosure

The message of so many books about dental practice, including this one, can be reduced to a simple statement: "It's important to build good relationships with your patients." The question comes when we wonder how to do it. It's similar when "experts" tell me to eat a diet balanced in proteins, carbohydrates, and fats. My typical response is, "Sounds good, but how do I do it?"

Disclosure is the essence of building relationships. Before defining disclosure, however, let's look at primary and secondary audiences. When I speak to a dental association, my primary audience consists of dentists and team members. However, these same people also make up the secondary audience. Aside from being in the dental industry, they are also sons or daughters, parents, spouses, vegetarians, hockey players, musicians, and more. The same is true for me. My primary role is that of the dentist/speaker. My secondary role is that of parent, spouse, son, water-skier, musician, ballroom dancer, great lover, and more!

I cannot separate or ignore the secondary audience. Therefore, my goal as a speaker is to appeal to the primary *and* the secondary audience. I appeal to the primary audience through my primary role with my content, relevance, credibility, and experience as a dentist, which fall into the blue spectrum arena.

I appeal to the secondary audience by revealing the experiences of my secondary role of parent, spouse, and so forth, which fall into the red spectrum arena. Overall, *I have as much or more in common with my secondary audience as I do with the primary audience.* Most audiences expect to hear me talk about my primary role, but when I reveal the experiences from my secondary role, I find that audiences become much more open to my presentation. Why? Because now the audience and I have more in common. We are more like each other than they realized. This "like me" phenomenon brings us closer. The appeal of my secondary role to the secondary audience is called *disclosure* and is a strong red spectrum tool.

You must use disclosure in the dental office if you want to sell complete dentistry. Disclosure is primarily achieved through storytelling, which I discuss in chapter 6. When you talk with a patient, keep one ear open for opportunities to disclose. If he mentions something about his secondary self, a hobby for example, think about how can you disclose something you both have in common.

Disclosure is at the heart of building relationships. Your primary role as a dentist allows a very narrow source of disclosure, which include shared experiences. Yes, there are times when your experience as a dentist can have enormous appeal to patients, but for most patients your secondary role is a much richer source of emotional appeal and persuasion.

What is a relationship if it isn't the shared or complementary experiences, values, and beliefs among people?

Have you ever met a patient in a restaurant who starts a conversation with you and you find yourself becoming uneasy? If this has happened to you, chances are you're not sure how to deal with the secondary roles, that of diners out for the evening, you and the patient now share. You'd probably be more comfortable talking with a stranger because the only roles you share with that person are secondary ones.

When you meet new patients, most of them experience the same uneasiness you experienced in the restaurant, and for the same reason; they're not sure how to relate to you in your primary role. In addition, they're not sure how to act in *their* primary role. The solution? Let some of the secondary roles ease into your doctor-patient relationship through the technique of disclosure. You both will be more at ease with each other and you are planting the seeds of a great relationship.

Visual Language

The fourth component of being memorable and persuasive is using visual language. Visual language consists of words that produce a picture in the mind of the listener. Visual language appeals to the visual mind, which is a red spectrum experience. Over time, our language has evolved toward being more abstract, which in contrast to visual language, appeals to the logical mind, a blue spectrum experience.

For example, if I said that I have an object in my car that weighs 0.75 kilograms and is 1.0 cubic feet in volume (abstract blue spectrum language), what do you see in your mind? Probably nothing. But if I said I have something in my car that's about the size and weight of a loaf of bread (visual red spectrum language), you can grasp one aspect of the object.

Visual language includes stories, metaphors, similes, and colorful comparisons to things that the listener can easily see. You can't see 1.0 cubic feet (abstract), but you can see a loaf of bread (visual). When I say, "She has a beautiful smile," what do you see? But when I say, "Her eyes are as clear as the sky and her smile is bright as the sun," do you see more?

When you see more in your mind, you'll remember more. It's easier to remember pictures than abstract concepts, which are necessarily vague because of the limitation of that type of language. Which is easier to remember: "A house on 815 Poplar Avenue," or, "The big white house on the corner"? You can't see 815 Poplar, but you can see the big white house on the corner. When you want patients to remember a concept, use visual language and you can expect greater understanding and recall of your message.

Some abstract, blue spectrum words we use with patients every day include: "quality," "laminate veneers," "periodontal disease," "endodontics," "inflammation," "osseointergration," "tooth reduction." What do your patients see in their mind when you use these words? Probably nothing. Would they see more and remember more if you said "suitable," "front-tooth covering," "gum infection," "pulp therapy," "redness," "rock-solid in bone," "tooth reshaping"? So, do you need to use visual language in the dental office? You do if you want people to understand and remember your recommendations for complete dentistry.

If you want to be memorable and persuasive and sell complete dentistry, then use the red spectrum tools of expression. Use your *attitude* to let people know how excited and committed you are about doing complete dentistry. They'll become excited only if you are. Use your ability to *connect* with people and let them experience your full attention. This connection makes people feel important. Use *disclosure* to build the relationship. It's easy to do business with someone with whom you have things in common. Use *visual language* to make the many abstract things in dentistry come to life in your patient's mind and be retained there. ***What is remembered is sold.***

CHAPTER 6

The Story You Tell Will
MAKE THE DIFFERENCE
In WHO YOU
Become

StorySelling® in Dentistry

Stories are magic. Study any book about management, leadership, or selling, and you'll find all the authors agree that telling great stories to illustrate your ideas is critical to your success. All great past and present leaders, business professionals, salespeople, and managers use storytelling to distinguish themselves, their ideas, build relationships, and make great first impressions. You can, too.

Why is any business successful? It's successful because of the success of its customers. ***What is your practice if it isn't the success of your patients?*** But who is telling your patients' stories to the public and to new patients? Right now, probably no one. But you and your staff can change that by telling the success stories of your patients. If do not tell these stories, then you're missing the most compelling reason for people to get their teeth fixed, which in essence is the story of all the other people who have found help and hope for their dental problems. The story you tell will make the difference in who you become.

StorySelling®

When you combine your story with a business objective involving leadership, managing, or selling, *storytelling* becomes *StorySelling*. The Coca-Cola Company, Hallmark Cards, Apple Computer, Adobe Systems, Grocery Manufacturers of America, Nike, Pinnacle Systems, Intel, Silicon Graphics, Simon & Schuster, and many others are all masters in the art of StorySelling. The technique is becoming a powerful tool in the business world because it memorably and persuasively communicates. The concept of StorySelling includes narratives, colorful comparisons, metaphors, and similes. Moreover, StorySelling is one of the most powerful red spectrum tools you can use to lead, but not push, people toward the right decisions and behavior.

Why Tell Stories?

Why do stories work so well as a case acceptance tool? Stories are the natural medium to convey appealing messages. Stories are an ancient art form, and King Solomon was recognized as the wisest man in the world because he knew more stories (proverbs) than anyone else.

Many profound decisions, including decisions about dental health care, are made with a strong emotional influence. More than any other device, stories tap into emotions. Without stories, much of professional dental communication is a "data dump" of information that patients are unlikely to remember; it's forgettable blue spectrum material.

Consider the way your staff and patients understand, believe, and remember things. If they *understood* what you said, did they *believe* it? And if they believed it, did they *remember* it? And did they remember the *key things* that led them to the outcome you wanted? This is what stories can do.

Wash Your Hands

Let me give you a personal example. When I was in grade school, my mother reminded me again and again to wash my hands. Naturally I looked for ways not to, until one day she told me this story:

"The railroad switching yard was just down the street from the house I grew up in, and your grandpa would send us kids to the tracks early in the morning when the locomotives were switching cars. As the coal cars would slam against each other, coal would be jarred out of the hoppers onto the tracks. We'd run up the hill like ants, grab the coal with our little hands, pack it in paper sacks, and bring it back to our father.

"We were poor and we needed the coal to keep the kitchen warm. At school we could always tell who the poor kids were because their hands would be dirty from coal." Then my mother looked right at me and asked, "Do you want people to think we're poor?"

I'll never forget that story and forty years later I still remember to wash my hands. Notice that this wasn't just a story about my mother's childhood. No, this was a personal story tied directly to a management objective: persuading me to wash my hands.

Dr. Brian Spillman of Indianapolis, Indiana says, *"...we talk about educating patients, but I think we have it backwards; we should be talking about educating ourselves. We need to be educated about who this person is and what his or her frame of reference is. And then, instead of giving the person technical details, tell a story. Patients don't know what vertical dimension or occlusion means, but they understand us when we say: 'You remind me of a particular person...'"*

The heart of StorySelling is that it helps the listener, patients, and staff to see and feel your message. StorySelling is a leadership and selling tool that helps change behavior, whether it's to wash a pair of dirty hands, alter an attitude, or accept comprehensive care.

We remember what we feel more than what we hear.

Answering the Tough Questions

Here are the toughest questions in dentistry:

- "Why is this dentistry so expensive?"
- "Do I really need all this work?"
- "How much will this hurt?"
- "I'm not sure I should have this done—what do you think?"
- "Why won't you accept what my insurance pays?"
- "I don't have time to fix my teeth."

- "The bridge you did for me broke.
  What are you going to do about it?"
- "Why aren't you a provider for my new PPO?"

When you hear these questions do you find yourself groping for words, overexplaining things, or apologizing? My clients tend to find themselves answering these and other questions in the logical (blue) spectrum, the issue extensively discussed in chapter 4. But does logic effectively persuade a patient who is emotionally upset?

Here's a scenario:

"Oh, doctor, I'm scared to death about you grinding my front teeth down. Is it bad?"

"Don't worry, Mrs. Salvin. We'll use intravenous sedation for you. We use a combination of Versed and Inapsine. We'll monitor your vital signs every step of the way. You'll be fine!"

Does this answer relieve her? It might get the question swept under the carpet, but it does not ease her fear. Emotional issues in dentistry, including fear, pain, money, time, safety, beauty, and so forth, are not adequately addressed in the logical spectrum. Emotional issues are best addressed in the emotional spectrum, with support, when needed, from the logical spectrum.

The language tool of choice in the emotional spectrum is the story or story-like device.

How Stories Work

You're sitting around with your friends and someone starts telling a joke. *"A priest, a rabbi, and a dentist were on an airplane, when..."* Halfway through the joke you are reminded of another joke, and this process continues until everyone runs out of jokes.

So, why does this process work? It works because other people's jokes remind us of ours. The same is true for stories. My story will remind you of your story. The power of the story is the moment when my story reminds you of your story and we grow closer as a result.

Storytelling is a wonderful way we disclose information. My story reminds you of your story, and then, just like the joke-telling session, you'll tell me your story. Will your story provide me with information I could not have obtained on my three-page patient history form? You bet. You and I have more in common and we have a more personal relationship as a result of storytelling. Do you want your recommendations for care to be important to your patients? Help the patient develop a personal relationship with you and, consequently, the patient will feel connected to the dentistry the patient needs. Stories do that.

**When things become personal,
they become important.**

Story Structure

Here's a simple structure and sequence for storytelling that has worked for centuries. It comes from Donald Davis, a master storyteller. It looks like this:

FIGURE 1: Story structure

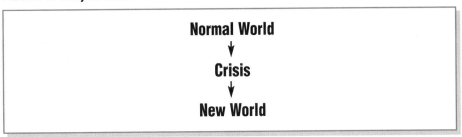

The *normal world* describes the world at the beginning of the story. "Once upon a time…" signals the description of the normal world. In the classic story of *Cinderella*, the young girl's normal world consisted of doing housework all day and suffering under the rule of her three nasty stepsisters and her evil stepmother.

The *crisis* of the story is the event that changes the normal world. "Then one day…" signals the arrival of the crisis. In *Cinderella* the crisis occurs when her tiny foot slipped into the glass slipper. As you can see, the crisis does not necessarily mean something bad. In terms of story, any life-changing event is a crisis: big promotions, weddings, divorces, the birth of a first baby, finishing dental school, and so on.

The *new world* is the way the world looks following the crisis. In Cinderella's case we don't know much about her **new world** other than she married the prince, moved into his castle, and, of course, "lived happily ever after."

To use stories effectively in a business setting or in the dental office, the story must have a point, an important reason for telling it. Unlike traditional storytelling, which is an entertainment art, StorySelling in a business setting teaches or persuades your listener. The teaching and persuasion components of StorySelling come from lessons learned during, or resulting from, the crisis. The lessons form the reason to tell the story; a lesson is transferred to the listener and it can then become the listener's lesson. StorySelling is a great way to tell people what to do without triggering anger. Here's how this looks:

FIGURE 2: StorySelling Structure

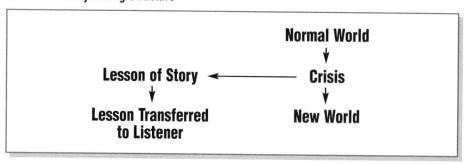

Aesop's fables always contained a lesson for the reader, which we have come to call the moral of the story. These were simple stories whose characters experienced crises. The lessons gained from these crises were transferred to the reader, implying that if the character in this story had this crisis, you can have it, too. And what about the lessons the characters learned? You can learn them, too. And we can all "live happily...."

Using Stories in the Dental Office

Patients often ask why dental care is so expensive. How do you answer the "fee" questions? You may begin re-explaining your recommendations, emphasizing the care, skill, quality, and judgment involved in the process. Then you cross your fingers, a blue spectrum response. Like most of my clients you may respond to the "Why is it so expensive?" question in the logical spectrum. This is not an incorrect response, but it is an incomplete one.

Questions about fees and the "it costs so much" laments occupy the *emotional* spectrum. Most questions about money are emotional questions. Sure, your patients intellectually and logically understand what 10,000 dollars literally means. What they don't understand is how they're going to pay for the care, how much they may have to tighten their belt, and why they let their teeth get into this mess in the first place. These are all emotional, red spectrum, concerns. Here's a simple formula to address this question and many other emotional spectrum questions:

FIGURE 3: StorySelling Formula

- Think of a patient who had the same or similar question/objection but overcame it and successfully completed her dentistry.

- Recount the patient's **normal world** prior to having her teeth fixed.

- Recall the specific event (**crisis**) that motivated her to seek dental care.

- Describe her **new world** with new dental health.

- What **lesson** did this patient learn from her experience?

- How can this lesson be **transferred to the patient** you're talking to?

Notice that I've put the story structure in bold type. Let's put this formula to work with the question/objection: "Why is it so expensive?"

Think of a patient who had the same or similar question/objection, but overcame it and successfully completed his or her dentistry in this case *her* dentistry.

This patient reminds me of Mabel Aker.

Recount the patient's normal world prior to having her teeth fixed.

Mabel was recently divorced and scared to face the world. She had neglected her teeth, and felt guilty and embarrassed about it. Money had always been the reason for not getting her teeth fixed.

Recall the specific event (crisis) that motivated her to seek dental care.

Mabel's friends talked her into going out for dinner and dancing. She was pleasantly surprised by the amount of fun she was having. In the ladies' room while putting on lipstick, she noticed the plastic front tooth on her partial denture was loose and ready to fall out. She ran out of the restaurant in tears and knew then she had to do something about her teeth.

Describe her new world with new dental health.

Today, Mabel is a different woman. She laughs without worrying that her teeth look bad, and her kids love their "new" mom. She loves her new teeth and that makes Mabel feel good about herself, which makes life fun again.

What lesson did this patient learn from her experience?

Mabel learned the cost of poor dental health was greater than the cost to fix her teeth. Mabel's only regret is that she didn't have her dental problems taken care of sooner.

How can this lesson be transferred to the patient you're talking to?

The cost of poor dental health is greater than the cost to fix teeth. When we're finished with your care, you'll wish you had done it sooner.

Now you're ready. You're in the consultation room explaining treatment and fees to Kristen, who raises the concern about the cost. *"Why is it so expensive?"* she asks.

"I am asked that all the time, Kristen. You remind me of Mabel. Mabel hated the way her teeth looked and the way it made her feel about herself. She was concerned about cost, too.

"During an evening on the town with her girlfriends, Mabel's plastic front tooth on her partial denture loosened and almost fell off. That was the evening she decided to get her teeth fixed.

"Today, Mabel loves her teeth and loves how good she feels again. Her only regret is that she didn't do it sooner. You'll feel the same way, Kristen."

This story takes only seconds to tell and fits into the flow of the conversation. Does this story use the logical spectrum to answer the question: "Why is it so expensive?" It doesn't, because a logical response would be an explanation of lab fees, time, care, skill, judgment, overhead, and who knows what else. The logical response is not wrong, but it is incomplete.

Mabel's story doesn't do anything about the cost, but it demonstrates how others eliminated or overcame the frustration and lived "happily ever after." And if other people can do it, so can she.

Using stories broadens our expressive range—our appeal.

The stories in your resource inventory broaden your expressive range and make you a more influential and memorable communicator. In the real world of dentistry, neither logical or emotional spectrum responses will overcome, answer, or acknowledge every concern. By themselves logical and emotional responses are both incomplete.

Here is a comment I hear a lot when I teach StorySelling: "Stories sound good, but you're not answering the patients question. It's like you're talking around their complaints."

Stories are one part of the process of responding to patients and by their nature, stories occupy the red spectrum. Many dentists believe that patient concerns should be answered in the blue—logical—spectrum. This is neither true nor even possible. Many of the greatest concerns patients have cannot be relieved or completely answered with logic. "I'm afraid," "I don't know where I'll get the money," "How will I look when I'm all done?" or "How do I know that I'll be happy with all this dentistry?" are expressions of frustration and concern rather than objections. Stories are excellent tools to acknowledge and ease frustrations and laments.

Patient frustrations are much like your response when you're ready to go to the beach and it's cold and raining. You may say, "Why is it raining?" And your know-it-all spouse might say: "Well, the dew point has been high and with that cold front coming through, I'm not surprised we experienced condensation, cumulous cloud formation, and consequently, precipitation."

It's the logical answer, but does this ease your frustration? No, it irritates you. But, what if your spouse reminded you about the time rain ruined the beach trip, and you went to the mountains, found a little cozy cabin, bought some wine and cheese, and had a lovely romantic weekend? It doesn't do anything about the rain, but the story works wonders for your frustration.

> **Telling patients you'll work within their budget doesn't do anything about the fee, but it can do wonders for their frustration.**

Your StorySelling® Inventory

I've found that creating a story inventory is a remarkably valuable process for selling complete dentistry. Here's how to create your story inventory:

> • Make a list of all the tough questions, objections, and comments you hear that relate to patient acceptance of complete dentistry. You'll find that there are about eight to ten questions or objections you'll hear on a consistent basis. They'll all be red spectrum concerns.

• Make a list of patients who had similar concerns but overcame them, completed treatment, and are happy they did. Match this list to the list of tough questions.

• Discover what the patient's **normal world, crisis,** and **new world** look like, and what lessons the patient learned.

Patients will disclose their normal world in terms of their chief complaint: "I hate the way I look," "I can't chew," "I hate dentists," "I'm in pain." Get a little deeper into their chief complaint and ask how poor appearance, fear, inability to eat, and pain affected their life. Listen carefully, because what you'll hear is a description of their normal world.

Patients occasionally will disclose their crises. Ask if there was a specific event that influenced them to make the appointment with you. Most patients will not eagerly or easily volunteer this information because it's often embarrassing and they're not sure you're the one to help them yet.

Rarely are dental teams aware of the patient's **new world** and **lessons**, and this is the step many of my clients find the most difficult. Sometimes patients forget the event that pushed them over the edge and made them ready for dental care. You'll find that patients are much more eager to talk about their **crises** and **lessons** when treatment is complete and they've had some time to enjoy their dentistry and grow in their appreciation of you. Dental teams find it easier to talk to patients about their lessons and crises after the first recall appointment.

Talking about a patient's **crisis** and **lessons** may seem awkward at first. Persevere, however, knowing that its the **crisis** and **lesson** that form the heart of the reasons that your new patients can say yes to complete dentistry. To continue the process:

- Put the patients from your list into the story structure.
- Practice these stories at staff meetings. When you've got the stories polished and can deliver them in under fifteen seconds, audio record them so everyone on the team can learn them while they're driving. It's important that everyone on the team is ready to tell a great story. "Golden Moments" are great opportunities for StorySelling. (You'll learn about them in chapters 14 and 15.)

Great stories are the "silver bullets" for responses to the tough questions. You already know what the patient's objections will be to your recommendations for complete dentistry. You've already learned your logical responses. Now it's time to learn your emotional responses and communicate over the entire range of appeal. Will your stories overcome or acknowledge every objection? No, they won't. Have your logical responses overcome every objection? No, they haven't. Together, logical and emotional responses will give you the most persuasive and memorable communication style, which is exactly what you need if you want to sell complete dentistry.

The Most Important Story to Tell

The most important story to tell illustrates why you practice dentistry—"YourStory." If you're a staff member, the most important story to tell illustrates why you work for your dentist. YourStory is the mother of all stories and is used as the answer to a wide variety of issues, including case acceptance, patient management, and objections. Its impact results from the fact that it discloses your beliefs. Those beliefs are illustrated and then offered to the patient as a reason (belief) for them to accept your recommendations.

I used my story for twenty years. My dental history is dramatic. I developed a slanting open bite with a full centimeter anterior open bite. As an adult the only teeth that made contact were my second molars. My speech and chewing were difficult. In 1975 I endured extractions, orthodontics, palatal expansion, vertical pull chin cup, head gear, and a sagital split osteotomy. I know what it's like to have bad teeth and I know what it's like to get them fixed. I use my story to answer the tough questions about pain, cost, time, and value.

For example, Kate, one of my young patients, asked if she really needed all the work I recommended. I answered her by telling her a short version of my story.

"Kate, twenty-five years ago I had teeth that were much worse than yours. I was a junior in dental school when I decided to get them fixed. Now I love how my teeth look and feel. I'm glad I had them fixed when I was young. You'll be glad, too."

You may not have dramatic dental history to share, but you can tell your patients how you feel about dentistry and how you enjoy seeing great results. You can talk about how you love helping people and why you want to make a difference in people's lives. Then transfer your belief to the patient: "You'll see great results, too," "I'll enjoy helping you," "This dentistry will make a difference in your life."

Notice that the story I shared with Kate consists of only five sentences. Each sentence coincides with the story structure: **normal world, crisis, new world, lesson, transfer lesson to the listener.** Most stories can be told in five sentences. Work on them until you have them down to the simplest language with the fewest words.

Good short stories are more persuasive and memorable than long boring ones.

Your staff members need to tell patients why they work for you, and the formula for the story is the same. Use the reason your staff works for you as the reason patients should have their teeth fixed. For example, your patient Guy tells your assistant Sally that he's worried about costs. She then says:

"Guy, I've been a dental assistant for eight years and have worked in three other offices. I love dental assisting and wanted to find an office that appreciated me. I've been here now for five years and I feel great about working here. They take good care of people here and they'll take great care of you, too."

The best story I've heard from a staff member is told by a hygienist in the office of Dr. John Hopp in Gillette, Wyoming. I challenged her to tell me a story that would convince me to have my teeth fixed. She didn't hesitate a second. She said:

"Paul, you remind me of my father. My mom and dad became patients in this practice fifteen years ago. They both had dental

problems like you do—loose teeth and infected gums. My mom went through treatment and today she has all her teeth. My dad didn't and today he wears dentures. What would you like to do?"

Top that story! Here's how to structure YourStory (dentist or staff member):

FIGURE 4: Your story.

- Reconstruct your normal world before you became a dentist or worked for your dentist.
- Recall a crisis that changed the way you relate to dentistry.
- Describe how this created your new world.
- What lesson did you learn from this experience?
- How can this lesson be transferred to the patient you're talking to?

Stories have powerful influence. Learn to tell them in short conversational language. Stories help you acknowledge the toughest issues and emotions, and the success stories of your practice define your practice. Stories create appeal, which leads to case acceptance, and indeed, the stories you tell make the difference in who you become.

CHAPTER 7

Don't Train the Horse, TRAIN THE Rider

The Philosophy of Complete Dentistry Case Acceptance

Brace yourself. It's time to challenge some time-honored philosophies of case acceptance. Over the last two decades, the clinical and diagnostic tools of dentistry have evolved rapidly, but many traditional techniques for case acceptance have not adapted at the same rate. What we did in the past was not wrong, but what worked well for traditional tooth dentistry does not work well at the complete care level. It's time to rock the boat and examine new philosophies for case acceptance of complete care. So start paddling.

Case acceptance for complete dentistry is not about changing patients. It's about changing ourselves. We like to blame our troubles on insurance companies, the patients, or your staff. It's easier to look outside ourselves when we face current challenges in our profession. However, the first person to look at when a patient says no is the one in the mirror. If you don't like what's going on in your life, don't try to change the world, change yourself.

My wife, Carolyn, rides dressage. You may have seen dressage on television. The horse and rider do intricate movements and the rider directs the horse with imperceptible leg and hand pressure. It's beautiful to watch and nearly impossible to do.

I asked my wife how she trained the horse to do all those unnatural movements. "None of the movements are unnatural for the horse," she said. "They all can be done by a horse in the wild without the rider."

"Well, how do you get them to do it when you want. How do you train the horse?"

"You don't train the horse, you train the rider," she said.

Don't train the horse, train the rider. But what if we spend all our time training the horse? We could attempt to raise the horse's dressage IQ by having it watch dressage videos or by hanging around other dressage horses. We could always teach it to speak English so we could give a long lecture to it! Don't teach the horse to speak English, learn to speak horse.

**Don't make patients speak dentistry,
learn to speak patient.**

Four Parts

The philosophy of case acceptance for complete dentistry has four parts. This philosophy:

- Focuses on target patients.
- Builds value early.
- Knows the difference between quality and suitability.
- Understands why raising a patients' dental IQ may not make them ready for care.

In this chapter we examine the importance of focusing on target patients. In subsequent chapters we'll look at the other three parts of the philosophy.

Focus on Target Patients

The first thing I noticed when I walked into my new client's reception room was a close-up photograph of a smile. It was four feet long, just teeth and lips—no face. The picture was right above the couch, on the opposite wall. I couldn't miss it.

"Dr. Hart will be with you in a minute," the receptionist, Ginger, said, as she handed me their office brochure.

The brochure was first class, four colors and nice paper. It featured cosmetic care, implant dentistry, and pedodontic procedures. The brochure included copy about saving teeth with endodontics and had pictures of adolescents in braces, and the piece was topped off with facts about nitrous oxide, free parking, and Saturday hours.

At a staff meeting I asked the dentist and staff to describe their ideal patient in terms of the dentistry needed, the patient's age, and the typical fee.

"I like the implant prosthetic patient," said Dr. Hart, which earned him an odd look from his chair-side assistant, Cathy.

"I didn't know you wanted to do more implant work. All we ever talk about, it seems, is cosmetic care and crown and bridge," said Cathy.

"We're a family practice," the hygienist, Rose, said. "We treat the needs of the family. We don't go out of our way to create dentistry we want to do, we do what the patient needs. It doesn't make any difference if they're young or old. Our doctor is well trained and he is great with children as well as adults." Rose had been with the practice fifteen years and saw herself as the practice's historian and conscience.

"I like the patients who pay us," Ginger giggled, much to the obvious displeasure of Dr. Hart and Rose.

It was becoming clear why Dr. Hart had severe stress, high overhead, and low case acceptance in his practice. He and his staff did not share a clear vision of the patient they most wanted to treat. They focused equally on all patients, and over time they were burning out on the overload, the diversity of care, the insurance issues, and all the normal but unacceptable behavior of a widely divergent patient base. Dr. Hart needed to focus on the type of dentistry he most wanted to do, on the patients who most likely needed that care, and on a fee that would compensate his office well. Dr. Hart needed to identify his target patient.

Who is your target patient? To help you figure this out, complete the following statements:

1. The type of dentistry I enjoy doing and want to do more of is:

_____

2. The typical age range of patients who need this type of dentistry is: _____

3. The typical fee range associated with the dentistry I enjoy doing is: _____

Now combining your three answers, describe your target patient. Here are some typical target patients for many of my clients.

a. Implant/rehabilitative dentistry, 45- to 65 year-old women; typical fee, $5,000 to $10,000 or more.

b. Cosmetic dentistry, 25- to 45 year-old women/men; typical fee, $2,000 to $6,000.

c. Crown and bridge/operative, 20- to 50 year-old women/men; typical fee, $1,500 to $3,500.

How Many Target Patients Do You Have?

How many total active patients do you have in treatment now, meaning treatment in progress or in active re-care who are seen at least once a year? How many of these are target patients? If you're like most dentists, targeted patients comprise less than 15 percent of all patients. Examine figures 1-3. If we call the 15 percent "target patients," what label should we attach to the other 85 percent? How about "stuff"! The stuff in your practice is all of the treatment you do that may not be what you want to do. It's stuff. It's low-fee tooth dentistry stuff. *In most dental practices, the stuff competes for our focus.*

Tooth dentistry can distract us, like someone on a cell phone in a movie theater.

FIGURE 1: TARGET PATIENTS: What is your percentage of target patients?

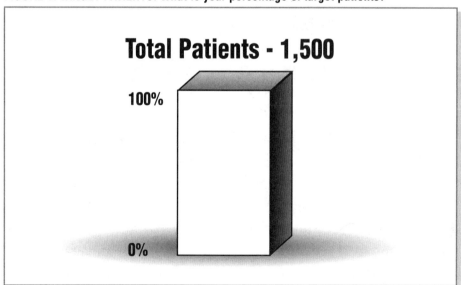

FIGURE 2: TARGET PATIENTS

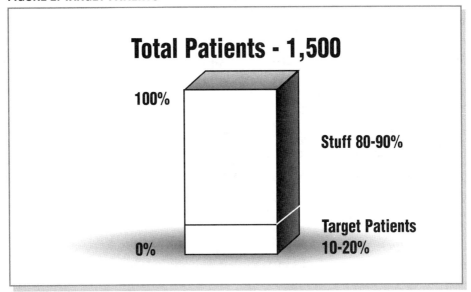

FIGURE 3: TARGET PATIENTS

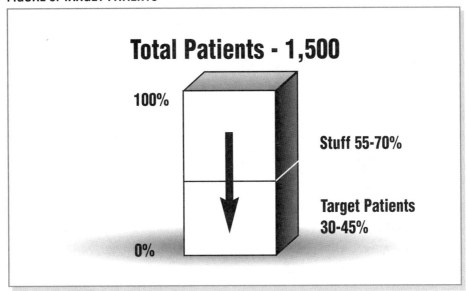

How much has stuff made its way into your practice? Your answers to the questions below are sure to clarify this issue for you.

1. What do you spend most of your time doing? Stuff? Target patients?
2. Who cancels appointments?
3. Who doesn't pay you?
4. Who hassles you about insurance?
5. Who complains the most?
6. Who are your office systems, i.e., scheduling, collections, insurance, and so forth designed to manage?
7. Who is your computer practice management software designed to manage?
8. Who does most of the practice management continuing education you've taken focus on?
9. Who brings you the greatest joy with respect to practicing dentistry?

If you're like most dentists I work with, your score is "stuff, 8" and "target patients, 1." Does this mean you need to get rid of the stuff? You better not, because that stuff can turn into target patients if you plant the right seeds and show these patients the way. It's been my experience that over three years, most general practitioners can enjoy a patient census that is 20 percent to 40 percent target patients by selling one to two complete care cases a month. After putting the ideas of this book into action, you can realistically set a goal of adding *one to two complete care cases a month.*

Identifying your target patient is important because it shapes the way you communicate your practice value to your patients and the public. Consider these solid reasons to identify your target patient:

- The concept of the target patient gives you an element around which to organize your facility. A facility that targets adults age forty-five to sixty-five should have a totally different look than a practice that targets children.

- Knowing your target patient will influence your continuing education decisions and equipment purchases.

- Being aware of your target patients sharpens your staff's ability to manage them, appeal to them, and have them refer others just like them.

- By knowing your target patient, your marketing can be developed to attract your target patient.

- By treating a higher percentage of target patients, you'll reduce the number of patients you see per day, your average treatment fee will increase, your overhead will decrease, and you'll experience less stress. *You'll actually have time to talk to people, especially your target patients.*

Identifying and attracting target patients does not mean you are going to treat them exclusively. For most general practitioners, it's a big mistake to limit themselves to a narrow treatment range. The purpose of the target patient concept is to help refine and sharpen your practice, but not limit it. Most general practitioner dentists should continue to treat a variety of patients. The concept of the target patient will enable you to see more target patients over time and gradually refine your practice.

Some of the happiest and wealthiest dentists I know are "bread and butter" dentists. They treat 20 percent to 40 percent target patients, run a tight ship, are still married, and have a life outside of dentistry.

Compelled Target Patients

Compelled target patients are the ones who walk in and say, "I'm ready!" These are the individuals who have compelling motives for having their teeth fixed. The problem is that only a few are compelled; only a few are ready to get their teeth fixed. Our mistake is in trying to make patients ready through our lofty mission statements, elaborate case presentations, and high-tech patient education.

You can't force people to be ready. The more you try, the more you'll suffer. Instead, use your energy on attracting and identifying those who are ready—compelled.

Imagine yourself driving home on a rainy night. It's about midnight and as you come to a top of a hill on the interstate, you hit the brake because traffic is backed up for miles. You see two tractor-trailers turned over at the bottom of the hill and hundreds of red taillights glow from the cars inching by the wreck. For the next twenty minutes you creep toward the wreck and soon discover that the trucks in the accident are on the median and are not blocking traffic. The motorists inching by in their cars aren't blocked; they're looking at the accident! Of course, this makes you all steamed up and you wish everyone would speed up so you can get home. But when it's your turn to pass the accident, guess what you do? You slow down and look at it. You now find yourself doing the same thing that irritated you just a few minutes before. So, why did you slow down and look and the wreckage? *You're compelled to—you can't stop yourself.*

Now imagine this. You're a fifty-seven year-old wife and grandparent. Your kids are grown and have families of their own. When you were fifteen, an old-timer dentist told your parents that you had "soft teeth" and for your high school graduation present, you had all your teeth removed. You went to your senior prom with your first set of dentures.

Over the years you had new sets made and just recently your dentist told you that since so much bone had resorbed new dentures wouldn't help anymore. Because of your embarrassment, it's easy to find excuses not to meet friends for dinner or enjoy intimacy with your husband. The good times of your life are passing by you like a stranger in a crowd. You feel very old and alone.

One day you see an advertisement for implant and cosmetic dentistry. It talks about permanent tooth replacements and smile enhancements. You cut the ad out of the newspaper and immediately call for an appointment. Why do you call so quickly? You call because you're *compelled* to call—you can't stop yourself.

When patients are compelled to do something, there's little that will get in their way. Ask yourself: Do you offer dental services that your target patients are compelled to seek? How many of your new patients are compelled to be in your office? How can you tell if they're compelled? Here's a short quiz:

1. Have they traveled more than forty-five minutes to see you?
2. Are they age fifty or older?
3. Do they match the demographic of your target patient?
4. Have they admitted to having a significant dental disability?
5. Are they interested in being seen as soon as possible?

If your new patient matches these characteristics, chances are great that you have a target patient with a compelling reason to see you.

I remember the first time I met a patient who was compelled. His name was Bob, a jolly wine distributor in his thirties from Hickory, North Carolina. Bob had been totally edentulous since he was fifteen years old. Predictably, his mandible was moderately atrophic.

"I read in the newspaper that you do dental implants. That's what I want 'cause I hate this denture," Bob was quick to say.

I was twenty-seven years old and I had just finished taking my first course in implant dentistry. I had never placed an implant, I had no visual aids to show him, and no testimonials from other patients.

I looked him in the eye and said: "I recommend we do a Ramus Frame implant for you. The surgery takes about two hours and we do it right in the office. I've never done one, so we'll fly to Florida and do it in the office of Dr. Harold Robbins. He's done hundreds. Afterwards, well come home and I'll build you new teeth. The total treatment fee is 4,600 dollars, which includes your airfare and lodging while we're in Florida. What do you think?"

"Great, when can we do it?" asked Bob.

Today, Bob is enjoying the twenty-third year of his implant.

How to Attract Compelled Target Patients

How did Bob find my practice? I had encouraged our small-town newspaper to write a small article about implant dentistry and Bob read it. If I hadn't participated in this article, I might still be waiting for Bob to show up. Thinking back on Bob and thousands of patients like him, I realize that appropriate and targeted marketing is a great way to help guide compelled patients to your door. *Because these patients are compelled, they will show up at someone's door, and your job is to show them the way to yours.*

I said earlier that less than 10 percent of new patients in the average dental practice are ready for complete dentistry. So if you have one candidate for complete dentistry this month, how do you treat one-tenth of a patient? You don't. However, if you have ten candidates for complete dentistry, chances are good that you'll end up treating one of them. One complete case a month, over time, will boost your practice enormously.

If you want greater case acceptance of complete dentistry, you need more patients who are ready for it to walk through your door. This means marketing your practice to attract compelled target patients.

You can attract many compelled target patients from outside your existing patient base. Most compelling dental conditions occur after men and women pass their fiftieth birthday, and these potential patients often don't know help is available. They silently suffer until something jolts them, such as the death of a spouse, a divorce, a promotion, or a wedding.

The secret to finding the compelled patient is to market to the deepest dental disability you and your treatment team are capable of treating. These disabilities include full and partial edentulism, severe dental phobia, and severe fear of tooth loss. You'll discover that when you attracted patients like these, all other areas of dentistry come along with this patient, including cosmetic procedures, TMJ, implants, and periodontics. Chapter 19 discusses the techniques of marketing to appeal to the compelled target patient.

How to Manage the Compelled Target Patient

Compelled target patients walk in ready for care, but most of them are not ready to choose you. Making that choice takes time. Remember our discussion of *emotional speed* from chapter 4? The biggest mistake we make is forgetting that while we're doing our examination, patients are doing theirs. And compelled target patients *do not* want to be disappointed with their examination.

Compelled patients want you to pay attention to them—they want you to connect. Too many of our tools for examination, the radiographs, periodontal probing, patient education videos, and so forth, can get in the way. Your flexibility during the new patient experience is the most important difference between dealing with compelled patients and dealing with stuff.

With your target patients, spend your energy and time making a good first impression. The temptation is to focus on blue spectrum activities: the complete examination, diagnostic procedures, and discussions about treatment options. In succeeding chapters you'll learn to minimize clinical procedures at the initial experience and focus on:

- Listening to the patient's story (chapter 6)
- Doing a simple overview examination (chapter 13)
- Discovering the basis for the patients' emotional distress with their oral health (chapter 13)
- Making them right (chapter 14)
- Having you and your staff tell stories of how you've treat-ed   many people just like them (chapter 14)
- Immediately repairing chief complaints that create pain, poor appearance, or poor speech (chapter 13)
- Assuring them that you'll work within their budget (chapter 14)

The focus on target patients is meant to refine, not limit, your practice. Often treating only 10 percent to 20 percent more target patients boosts your profitability and morale to such an extent that the emotional climate of your practice changes and has new energy everyone can sense. You'll appreciate your patients more and be more apt to demonstrate your gratitude. And it's your appreciation and gratitude for the people around you that will boost your case acceptance for complete dentistry.

CHAPTER 8

What You Can LEARN At Your Bakery

Building Value

Why does the baker add an extra doughnut to your dozen? You order a dozen doughnuts, but you walk away with thirteen, the proverbial "baker's dozen." Your baker knows it's easier to give away one doughnut than to find another customer. The extra doughnut represents an unexpected positive experience, going the extra mile, and getting more than your money's worth. In a word, the doughnut is value. Complete care patients want and expect value.

One of the best examples of value I've seen occurred at a seminar I gave. The program was sponsored by Mark Marinbach, owner of Nu-Life Dental Laboratory in New York, and just before I started my program, Mark said, "Ladies and gentleman, please rise for the 'Star Spangled Banner.'" A young woman and man, both dressed in formal attire, walked to the front of the room. He sat at the grand piano, she picked up a microphone, and for the next five minutes the duo performed their rendition of the "Star Spangled Banner." It was a smash! They received a standing ovation and kicked off a program like I'd never before seen anyone do.

Mark Marinbach understands that value needs to be obvious, overwhelming, and immediate. He knows it's important to get a standing ovation *before* the program begins. Do you know how to get a standing ovation *before* your treatment begins? If you do, you're well on the way to selling complete dentistry.

The Timing of Value: Give Before You Get

Is there an optimum time to provide value? Would the "Star Spangled Banner" have been as effective at the end of the program? Based on my experience, value offered before treatment recommendations are made enhance their acceptance.

Doesn't it make perfect sense to build value early in the relationship to foreshadow the quality of experience during the treatment phase?

Here's a graph of traditional clinical thinking about value. I was taught, as were many of you, that patients have the greatest sense of appreciation and value *after* treatment is completed.

FIGURE 1: Traditional clinical thinking about value.

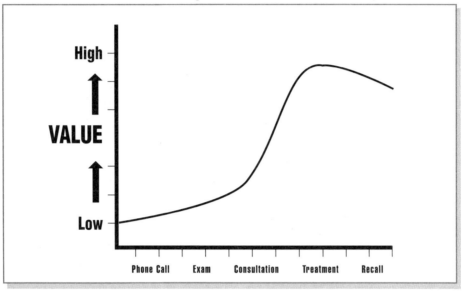

(Figure 1) In dentistry, it's customary to ask for referrals when care is *completed*. But what about patient "burnout?" Trust me on this. By the time they are done with a long series of appointments, the last thing they or any of their friends want to hear about is more dentistry.

Waiting to provide value and ask for referrals at the end of care is too late. Waiting to perform the "Star Spangled Banner" at the end of the program is too late.

FIGURE 2: The entrepreneurial perspective on value.

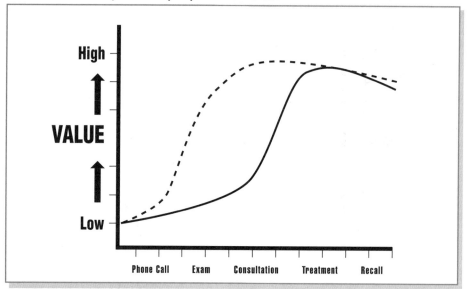

Look at the entrepreneurial perspective on value, which emphasizes maximizing it as soon as possible (Figure 2). In complete
care dentistry, providing value early:
- Enhances the acceptance of complete dentistry.
- Inspires patient referrals before and during the
  treatment process.
- Creates easier long-term patient management.

Enhanced Case Acceptance

Case acceptance for complete dentistry is enhanced when
patients have experienced value in your practice, and value is a
red spectrum experience. Dentists who are totally *clinically*
oriented, which means they stay in blue spectrum thinking, will
argue that the greatest value a patient can receive is superior

clinical quality. They believe the expectation of quality should be enough for patients to postpone their appetite for value now and wait for it to hit them at the completion of care. Does this sound familiar? Does this work?

The major flaw in this thinking is that clinical quality does not represent value. Value is a positive *unexpected* experience— getting more than your money's worth. The patient walks into your office expecting clinical quality. Isn't that what the patient is paying for? Saying the quality of your care is value is like a restaurant boasting that its food is digestible.

The greatest values in dentistry are found within relationships, not restorations.

Quality relationships are easily recognized by the patients, and create immediate and overwhelming responses. Plus, thanks to the societal stereotype of the dull dentist, a dentist (and staff) with great people skills is definitely a positive and *unexpected* experience.

Creating positive unexpected experiences—red spectrum—prior to providing care will do more for case acceptance than all of your promises of clinical excellence and adherence to quality.

[137]

Increase Patient Referrals

Providing value early gives you more opportunities for patient referrals. Patients are typically more excited and involved with the care before it starts than when it's finished. If you have been reconstructing your patient's mouth for nine months, she and everyone in her life, from co-workers to family members, are tired of hearing about her experiences. If you wait to ask for referrals at the end of treatment, her experience is already old news. No one cares and the last thing many of her friends want to hear is more about what she just went through. Instead, provide value early and ask for referrals early. *My experience has been that word of mouth is strongest before and during the treatment process.*

Long-term Patient Management

Early value makes long-term patient management easier. We're apt to forget about the smashed éclair in the box we bought last week if the baker gives us an extra doughnut today. The dental experience is laden with hassles, inconveniences, and expense. Early value helps take the sharp edges off some of the normal but unacceptable behaviors and events associated with dentistry. People will forgive us if they know our hearts are in the right place.

Rapport: Use It or Lose It

We always come back to rapport. Like you, your patients have met people they immediately liked or disliked, and they have had a similar experience when meeting you. The level to which you'll build your practice is dependent on your ability to build rapport. A dentist and team members with great personalities are an outstanding value to the patient.

Let's be clear. I'm not pitting standard of care, blue spectrum issues, versus personalities, red spectrum issues. But *patients* are making these comparisons all the time. Ask people what they like about their dentist. What do they say? They say, "She's good with children," "She listens to me," "He's gentle," "I like the staff," "It's an upbeat office," and "Everyone is so nice there." These statements reflect rapport, which is always a red spectrum issue.

Standard of care isn't the feature of value patients most respond to. You can prove this to yourself. Double what you believe to be clinical quality. Take every course you can on any clinical topic you'd like. Will you double your practice? No. For decades dentists have used the clinical quality approach to build their practices. As a result we have thousands of dentists who are terribly frustrated with their careers. They're well trained, but patients don't respond to their treatment plans. Many dentists are all dressed up with nowhere to go.

Now, try doubling your ability to build rapport and establish long term relationships. You'll find that the biggest payoffs in overall practice development, fulfillment, and referral base development are gained through rapport, which is a value issue. Go back to Daniel Goleman's quote in chapter 4 on academic versus emotional intelligence.

Incremental gains in rapport building far outperform incremental improvements in technical refinement.

Look in the Mirror

I know many dentists with unattractive teeth. If we want to chill our patients' enthusiasm for care all we need to do is have unattractive teeth. Patients look for signals of value. If you have perfectly matched crowns in your mouth they are excellent testimonies to the beauty of dentistry. The opposite is also true. Unattractive teeth provide a negative testimony. Would you take advice about your diet from an obese nutritional counselor or hire a personal trainer who's a chain smoker? Of course not! So why do so many dentists have unattractive teeth?

I had dinner with a young handsome specialist who complained he had trouble selling dentistry. His front teeth had a reverse smile line and were dark. I asked him if he'd considered having his teeth fixed. "I've thought about it but just haven't found the time," he replied. He sounded much like so many patients I've known. If you want to be perceived as a quality dentist and you want to provide value, then have pretty teeth.

You Don't Have a Fax Machine or E-mail?

Responsiveness is value. Do you know individuals who just can't be on time, follow through on tasks, or return telephone calls? What is the perceived value and quality of their work? We live in an accelerating world. Technology has made us impatient for results. At one time getting back to a customer with an estimate in a few days was fine. Our patients now live in a world in which the estimate must be faxed that day just to stay ahead of the competition. Pagers, e-mail, voice mail, faxes, computers, cellular telephones are all part of the everyday world of our patients. Are they part of yours?

Many dental offices still do not have fax machines or computers. Going into these dental offices is like taking a step back in time. Today, having a positive experience is next to impossible in an office that makes communication next to impossible, and by current standards "next to impossible" means: no fax, no e-mail, constant busy signals, and so forth.

> If we want to irritate a contemporary business or professional person all we need to do is have too few telephone lines, no e-mail, and answering machines that don't accept messages.
> If we are generally unreachable, eventually no one will try.

Do you really *want* to sell complete dentistry? Do you want to stay out of managed care and keep your patients from leaving and enrolling in an HMO? I assume your answer is yes to these questions, so make sure you join the twenty-first century and make it easy for your patients to communicate with you and easy for you to respond. The ability to reach your office and receive a fast response is an important *value issue* you cannot afford to overlook.

Throughout this book I'll give additional examples of how to build value. Create value that's obvious, overwhelming, and immediate. Get your standing ovation *before* your dentistry begins.

CHAPTER 9

Would You Rather Be
HAPPY or
Right?

The Difference Between
Quality and Suitability

Traditional thinking says the best way to gain case acceptance for complete dentistry is to improve our clinical quality, educate patients to recognize good dentistry, and both show and tell them the benefits of fine dentistry. Traditional thinking says the promise of quality is the *right* reason for patients to buy. But *happy* dentists benefit from knowing that patients buy for many reasons, some of which have nothing to do with quality. Would you rather be right or happy?

The Perpetual Argument

Many dentists argue that quality speaks for itself and sells itself. Most of these dentists are unhappy because they are unaware of an important distinction between quality and suitability. The dentist and staff revel in the *quality* of their work; they *know* the job has been exquisitely done. Patients relish the *suitability* of your work when they believe you have fulfilled their wants and needs well. Knowing the difference between quality and suitability is a key ingredient for selling complete dentistry.

Years ago I did a program at the Westin Inn in Winnipeg, Canada. I like to order room service breakfast so I can rehearse my stories. My only consistent complaint about most room service breakfasts is that the toast is always too cool to melt the butter. It's hard to keep toast warm on its trip from the kitchen.

I requested breakfast at 6:30 and the knock on the door was right on time. The server was a tall bellman with a big grin. His red hair was sticking straight up—like ironed ketchup. He waltzed in, tray balanced on his arm, and asked with a twinkle in his eye, "And what kind of day are we going to have today?"

I thought, "Hey, fella, lighten up, I'm the speaker!" But I said, "I'm going to have a great day."

"Well, every great day starts with a great breakfast."

And with flair he flipped out the tray stand, put the breakfast tray down, and lifted its dome covers. Then, without a word, he reached into a canvas bag on the side of the tray, pulled out a shiny toaster, put in two pieces of rye bread, pushed the toaster handle down, and said, "Have a great day." Like the Lone Ranger, he was out the door and disappeared.

The Westin Inn understands that suitable toast must be warm toast. I assumed the bread would be quality bread—no roaches, digestible, meeting all the requirements to get the Good Housekeeping Seal of Approval. But *suitability* means warm toast. Quality means FDA-approved toast. *Suitability is what the diner expects from a meal; quality is what the baker tries to deliver. Suitability is what the patient wants, quality is what the dentist and staff pursue. Suitability* is red spectrum, *quality* is blue spectrum.

FIGURE 1: Suitability is red spectrum, quality is blue spectrum.

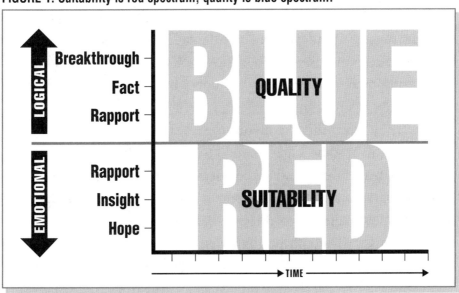

Suitability is the patient's experience; quality is the dentist and team's experience.

Suitability Close to Home

When my son Adam graduated from college, he called me and asked me where he could get his teeth cleaned. I recommended Dr. Jerry, a dentist not far from Adam's home. "He's a good guy," I said. "You'll like him."

I called his office, told him my son needed his teeth cleaned, and gave his receptionist my credit card number. Two weeks later I called Adam and asked about his dental appointment.

"They didn't clean my teeth," Adam said. "They talked to me for twenty minutes about my dental history, then I watched a video on gum disease. Then they took a ton of x-rays and molds of my mouth. When we were done, he asked me what I didn't like about my smile."

"They never did clean your teeth?" I asked.

"No, instead he said I needed to see an orthodontist."

I called Dr. Jerry and asked why he didn't clean my son's teeth. "We give all our new patients a quality experience," he said. "All new patients go through dental and health history, smile analysis, full-mouth radiographs, study models, face bow, and complete examination."

So, did my son receive quality dentistry? Some dentists would say yes, others would say no. An easier question, "Did my son receive suitable dentistry?" The answer is clearly no.

This anecdote raises numerous questions: If my son had been a compelled target patient who wanted to have his teeth cleaned, what would his opinion of Dr. Jerry's office be? Was my son happy with Dr. Jerry? Would he refer his friends to Dr. Jerry? Would he feel good about paying his fee? Would he be impressed? Would he have gained value—an unexpected bonus? Does my son's experience happen in your office?

What Are the Qualities of Quality?

For our purposes here, think of quality as a feeling, rather than a technical characteristic of your work. When you place a three-unit bridge and it snaps in to place, the contacts are snug, the color right on, and the occlusion perfect, how do you feel? That's what I call quality—how you feel about your work. It's as if you have a candle next to your heart. And when you do something technically spectacular, the candle flame surges and warms and comforts you. Quality for the *dentist and team* can be a red spectrum experience.

The difference between quality and suitability became clear to me years ago. I had just finished enjoying a mountaintop, snap-in-the-bridge experience. It was perfect!

"How do you like it?" I asked Lilly as I handed the mirror to her, fully expecting high praise and gratitude.

She glanced in the mirror, looked at the bridge for one second, then looked at her hair, groomed her bangs, smiled at me, and said, "It's fine."

That was the day I learned that my experience of quality is not the same as the patient's.

How Suitable Is Suitability?

Suitability is what the patient hopes for. Suitability is a red spectrum experience for the patient. Suitable experiences for the patient include:

- Fees within their budget
- Gentle touch, painless injections, absence of discomfort
- Appointments that fit into their schedules
- Quick and lasting results
- Dentistry that looks and feels good
- Respect
- Friendly and attractive dentist and staff
- Being seen on time
- Ethical behavior
- Sense of humor
- No pressure

What the patient finds suitable is not the same as what we deem to be quality. In fact, we may do a wonderful restoration (high quality) and the patient may have an awful experience (unsuitable), or do an awful restoration and have a patient as happy as a clam. Higher fee complete care patients, to a great extent, are purchasing suitability more than their lower fee tooth dentistry counterparts.

Kathy, a chair-side assistant at Dr. Timothy Droege's office, says, *"We used to spend too much time on the quality issue— telling patients why they should come back. 'Suitability' is a new word around here now. We concentrate on things patients appreciate, not what we think they need to hear."*

> **People expect more (suitability)
> from their dentist when their fee
> is $10,000, than at $850.
> You would, too.**

Mission Statements

I often see mission statements on the walls in my clients' offices. These statements usually highlight the dentists' attitude about the technical quality of the dentistry. But most are composed as blue spectrum statements. Many of them read like this:

"We strive to provide the finest quality dentistry to all our patients and restore their teeth to the highest level of function, comfort, and aesthetics. We perpetually educate and reinforce to all our patients the importance of preventative dentistry. We provide the highest possible level of clinical excellence in an environment that is safe, comfortable, and conducive to continued optimal oral health—so help us God."

This statement looks good in a frame, but how does it relate to suitability? Do all patients want the finest quality dentistry? Or do they want appropriate care (suitable care) based on their budget and schedule? Do all your patients expect or want the highest levels of function, or do they just want to chew comfortably? Are all your patients interested in being perpetually reminded of preventative dentistry? Frankly, who is?

I agree that a mission statement is a great management tool to clarify the vision for dentist and staff. But don't expect your patients to want, need, or appreciate your ideals. Don't assume quality leads to suitability.

In their zealous pursuit of excellence, many dentists leave their patients behind.

The Patient's Mission Statement

Patients have a mission statement, too. They may not have it framed, but they know it by heart, and it is always a red spectrum statement:

"I'll get my teeth fixed when I'm ready and when I can afford it. I want it done fast, painlessly, and I want it to look and feel great. I want it to be convenient and done by cheerful, attractive people."

If you want to sell more complete dentistry, build your mission statement around the patient's goals and attitudes. Don't confuse your pursuit of quality with the patient's expectation of suitability.

Logically, we want patients to accept dentistry on the basis of clinical quality because it is the component of care over which we have the most control and it's what we've been trained to do. Patients, however, have no control over quality and they make decisions based on what they understand, which are the suitability issues.

When you understand that patients buy dentistry for their reasons, not yours, everyone is happy. Would you rather be right or happy?

CHAPTER 10

When the
PATIENT IS READY,
The Dentist Will
Appear

Dental IQ vs. Patient Readiness

Patients get their teeth fixed when they're ready, and no sooner than that. If patients aren't ready and have many other things happening in their lives, your dentistry is going to take a backseat. If you push patients into care you'll just annoy them and waste time. In North Carolina there's an old saying: "Never try to teach a pig to sing. You'll waste your time, and irritate the pig."

If you believe complete dentistry is sold on the basis of your patients' understanding of what clinical quality is, then it makes perfect sense to educate them. Raise your patients' dental IQ so they can understand, appreciate, and want complete dental care.

But does this approach work? Is education a strong motivator and does it create an appetite for dentistry? It's been my experience that when my clients extend enormous effort to raise patients' dental IQ through elaborate case presentations, multimedia visual aids, and long and in-depth oral hygiene instructions, they and their staffs are often disappointed and waste everyone's time. Raising the dental IQ is not a prime motivator for case acceptance for complete care. The prime motivator is readiness. When the patient is ready, the dentist will appear.

Readiness has very little to do with what happens in your office.

Readiness is most often associated with something that happens *outside* the office, such as a divorce, a marriage, a new job, or a crisis.

I smoked for twenty years. I'd keep a pack of Kool Milds stashed in the glove compartment of my car, and after work I'd burn a few. Not many, maybe a pack or so a month.

One day in 1996 I had a complete physical examination from my family physician, Dr. Charles Furree, including a 12 lead ECG. As I was putting my shirt back on, Dr. Furree walked into the room. While looking at my record, he said the words you never want to hear following an ECG.

"I don't want to worry you, but…"

"But what?" I asked.

"You have atrial fibrillation. It's an irregular heartbeat—an arrhythmia."

"So what do we do about it?" I asked, hoping for the best.

"I'm referring you to Dr. David Framm. He's a cardiologist and I want him to do an echo ECG now."

"You don't understand," I said. "I'm booked to do a program."

"You don't understand," he said, "you're going now."

I went.

I got to Dr. Framm's office and after an examination and the echo ECG he confirmed the diagnosis of arrhythmia.

"So what's the cure," I asked.

"This is a common problem," he replied, "and the treatment involves hospitalization, drug therapy for three days, and on the morning of the third day, we'll cardiovert you."

"What does cardiovert mean?" I feared I knew.

"Oh, you know what that is. That's when we use defibrillator paddles on your chest and shock your heart back into normal sinus rhythm."

His words seem casual and controlled, while I had visions of my body bouncing three feet off the table as lightning bolts arced through it. A week later I was admitted to Carolinas Medical Center. They put me on medication and I lay in bed for three days waiting for my cardioversion. I had my notebook computer with me, got on line, and researched articles on atrial fibrillation, heart disease, and the afterlife. Do you know how many references to smoking are made in articles on heart disease? A whole lot! Did I know that smoking has health hazards? Yes! Did all the education on the hazards of smoking change my attitude about smoking? No. My cardioversion did.

Since that trip to the hospital, I haven't had a cigarette. Why? It wasn't because of education. It was the experience of being wheeled into the operating room, hooked up like an electric dryer, and waking up feeling like I had been kicked in the chest by a horse. I quit smoking—so would you.

At some point, all of us become ready for something. Maybe it's to lose weight, get married, get divorced, have a baby, or start saving money. Think back to a time that you knew what to do but weren't ready to do it. Then one day, you became ready, probably for a variety of reasons, some of which had nothing to do with the act itself. *Patients are just like you; they've had the same experience.*

Patients can have all of the reasons to get their teeth fixed paraded right in front of them; you can use all the logic in the world, and if they're not ready, the boat isn't going to leave the dock.

Growth Readiness

James Pride, DDS, founder of the Pride Institute, talks about the seven factors that contribute to the willingness to change, to grow. These factors are *passion, resourcefulness, optimism, adventurousness, adaptability, confidence,* and *tolerance of ambiguity.* These are all red spectrum factors. (See figure 1.) These factors create the *will* to grow. Will is a red spectrum experience. The will leads to action, and that's why we have the unforgettable adage: *Where there's a will, there's a way.*

Dentists are great at showing people the way. We love to tell people how we'll fix their teeth. But *the will must precede the way.* Telling complete care patients how to fix their teeth is showing them the way, but it often is not enough for them to find the will. Often they need to find the will on their own.

Dr. Tim Droege of Breeze, Illinois, says, *"I've learned not to waste my time trying to sell services to people who don't want them. We have a lot less stress in our office because we're not trying to convince everyone to do dentistry they're not ready for. It feels a lot better doing a procedure on people who have made a free choice about their dental work and don't feel pressured into it."*

FIGURE 1: Growth readiness

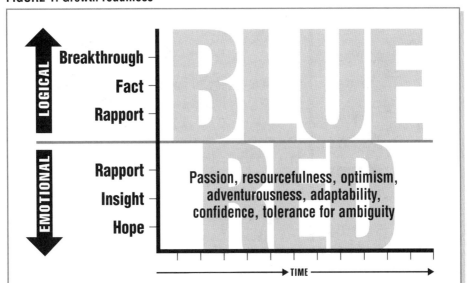

The old Zen proverb, "When the student is ready, the teacher will appear," applies to many things in life, and it most certainly applies to case acceptance. If you've ever tried to teach a skill to someone who wasn't ready to learn then you know exactly what I mean. If you've ever tried to sell someone a full mouth rehabilitation who wasn't ready for it, then you understand frustration. When your patients are ready, they'll tell you. (See figures 2, 3.)

**When the patient is ready,
the dentist will appear.**

FIGURE 2: Zen proverb

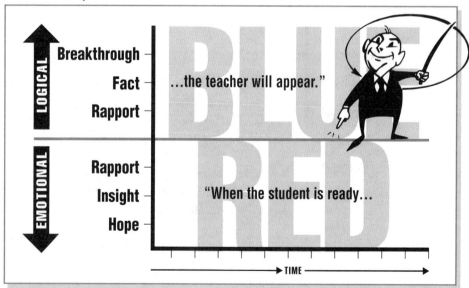

FIGURE 2: Dental proverb

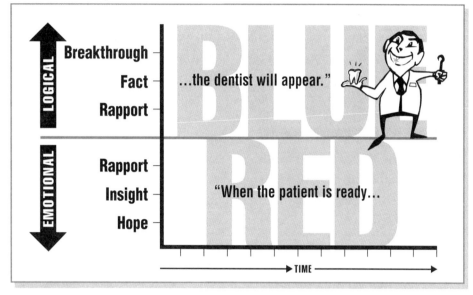

Ready or Not

Most patients are not ready for complete dentistry; in the average general practice, fewer than 10 percent of new patients are ready. We get into trouble when patients are not ready and we try to make them ready. We drag them through patient education videos, multiple hygiene visits designed to raise the dental IQ, and exhausting case presentations. Worse yet, we ask patients manipulative questions: "If I can show you a way to be happy with your teeth, is anything stopping you from making a commitment today?" Or "What don't you like about your smile?" These questions arise from the hope that patients will "cave in."

Since many of us want to practice complete dentistry, we put extra effort into making an appropriate candidate ready to want what we offer. We pour out our guts to them, we diagnosis and "treatment-plan" them through elaborate diagnostic tools, we educate them with the finest audiovisuals, and often when the smoke clears, our patient rolls her eyes and asks us to fix the front tooth and give her a new toothbrush. Another one bites the dust.

Making people ready is a great way to invite suffering into your career. Become good at saying "when you're ready…"

I encourage my clients to say, "when you're ready" before and after most treatment recommendations. For example:

"Adam, when you're ready, a good way to improve your chewing would be to replace your back teeth. I recommend we use permanent nonremovable teeth that you brush right in your mouth. The fee for your teeth is $2,500 and it will take us about one month from start to finish. Of course, we'd make sure that this fits within your budget and we'll start this when you're ready."

Impatient Education

When I teach the concept of readiness at a seminar, it always ignites controversy. I'll hear participants say something like: *"Yes, but isn't that what patient education is all about—helping people become ready. If we don't educate patients about what's possible, they'll never know that they can be helped. Besides, it's the educated patient, patients with the high dental IQ, who really appreciates their teeth and are the ones who'll opt for complete care."*

I don't oppose influencing patients and helping them understand and accept comprehensive care. I agree it is our responsibility to put dentistry's best foot forward. But there is a line between influencing and nagging that I see many dentists cross. *Influencing* is offering complete care. Influencing is having the right attitude and giving patients hope. Influencing is being willing to work within a patient's budget. Influencing is modeling you and your staff's excellent dental health. Influencing is having new patients talk with happy treated patients just like them.

On the other hand, *nagging* is forcing patients through long, expensive examinations and consultations when that isn't what they want. Nagging is criticizing them for poor dental health. Nagging is making subtle threats about the consequences of delayed treatment. Nagging is showing your disapproval of their financial limitations. Nagging is asking manipulative closing questions and using your position of authority to intimidate.

Where I differ significantly with many dentists who have a zealous, evangelistic attitude about dental health, is that I make it all right for someone with dental problems not to do anything about them, for now.

Dr. Joe Shae has changed his perspective on patient education. "We have backed off from a lot of the dental educational aids. I'm finding that I don't need them. I think that patient educational tools can scare people off more than motivating them. They don't understand crown margins or precision partial dentures. We'd hope that showing them a picture would inspire them to say yes. It didn't. Now we talk more about what patients want and what we offer, and we assure patients we can do the work within their budget. We tell them a story about somebody who has had similar work. And that's usually all we need for case acceptance.

"We've had some negative experiences with patient education tools. At one time we had a patient education video going continuously throughout the day. I don't know if you've ever seen the video of the spinning implant, where the gums open up, and the implant goes into the bone. I had a sweet older woman in here a little while ago. I was in the next room and the video came on and I heard her say, 'Oh, God! What is that?' I told the assistant to shut the video off – forever! I've had greater case acceptance of implants since I've stopped using the patient education video!"

Patients should never feel wrong for their position about care. I have found that when I don't make patients wrong, they return when they're ready. In addition, I don't make myself crazy wishing that patients would change!

Inform Before You Perform

You've heard this all your career and it's true: ***"Inform before you perform."*** Patients need to know what's going on. But be aware that "inform before you perform" is a consent issue, not an influencing technique. Don't confuse consent and influence. Early in our careers we didn't know about influencing. All we knew was consent and it was given after we informed. When patients said yes, we assumed they did because of our act of informing.

We get into trouble when we think that if a little informing sells low-fee tooth dentistry dentistry, then a lot of informing should work great at the complete care level. Put another way, the principle holds: *The more you perform, the more you should inform.* But this is not the way complete care dentistry works.

**Complete care requires more
influence than information.**

Do not confuse patient education and consent with influence. Patient education, consent, and influence overlap. Consent is the *information* that outlines the benefits, risks, and alternatives to care. Patient education provides *instruction* for patients to maintain dental health. Influence means *motivating* the patient to appreciate and want the benefits of care. (See figure 4.)

Patient education, consent, and influence include elements of each, but they have individual strengths, too: *consent informs, education instructs, influence motivates.* When dentists don't understand how to influence, they substitute information and

FIGURE 4: Consent and education vs. influence.

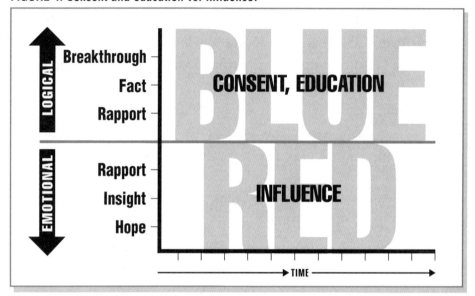

instruction and hope these elements will influence patients to accept complete care. Instruction and information are not substitutes for influence, just as influence is not a substitute for instruction or information.

To sell complete dentistry to your patients, you need to influence them. Dentists are trained in consent and patient education, but most of us are not trained in influence. Consequently, we offer a lot of information and education and hope it will change patients' behavior, that is, that they will then accept complete care. We must blend influence with consent and education to change behavior.

Most case presentations I see for complete dentistry are exaggerated forms of consent. But a lot of consent does not equal influence. Go back to the Spectrum of Appeal for guidance.

Informed consent and patient education are blue spectrum activities; influence is red spectrum.

Let Me Sell You the Solution

Based on my observations, adult patient education has evolved into a selling technique. The education process creates deficits, and in order to remove those deficits, there's a price. In *Dentists: An Endangered Species* I called this process: "You've got a problem, let me sell you the solution."

Imagine walking into a health food or fitness facility that offers fitness and diet screening for a reasonable fee. You'd like to be fit, so you decide to do it. The young hard-body saleswoman takes you through the fitness and examination process and lets you know you've got some *real problems*. You sense her disappointment when you can only do two pull-ups. You catch a certain edge to her tone of voice as she measures your body fat.

You hope the torture is over, but then she sits you down in front of a videotape, and for fifteen minutes you watch young athletes flex their muscles, all the while reminding you that this is not you. She takes a picture of you in your gym trucks and then uses a computer-imaging program to remove your love handles and tuck your tummy. "This is how a healthy body looks. Now what are you going to do about it?" chides Miss Hardbody.

Would you feel better or worse about yourself after this experience? Would this process raise your fitness IQ and make you want to be fit? How would you feel about the saleswoman? Would you be ready to plunk down your money to shut her up?

It seems that too much of dental patient education is a sales tool that has degraded to create deficits that weren't there when the patient walked into the office. And we're hoping patients will open their wallets just to shut us up.

Dr. Gayland Brown of Dixson, Tennessee talks about his experience with patient readiness:

"The main thing the principle of readiness did for our practice was to take away confrontation. Because I don't feel confrontational with the patients, they don't feel confronted. It took away the pressure of having to try to hard-sell dentistry. Let the patient arrive at that conclusion of what they need in their own good time. I stopped trying to herd people like a flock of geese and now allow them to decide when they're ready. It makes the relationships with my patients so much better and genuine. Patients sense that I'm interested in what they want. They believe we really care about them and are willing to work with them and not attempt to push them where we want them to go. Overeducating patients makes them feel pushed."

The Spectrum of Appeal

Let's put the issues of quality, suitability, dental IQ, readiness, and mission statements on the Spectrum of Appeal. (See figure 5.) Quality, dental IQ, and practice mission statements are logical, blue spectrum, issues. Suitably, readiness, and patient mission statements are emotional, red spectrum, issues. As

I said in prior chapters: for case acceptance for complete dentistry you need to use both spectrums, creating the broadest possible appeal.

No, *You* Change

Patient education attempts to get the patient to understand the fundamentals of dentistry and speak our language. We want to raise the patients' dental IQ to our level so they appreciate and want dentistry. We want them to change and think and do things our way. Think about that for a minute. How many people in your life have you changed? Think about your spouse, your teenagers, your patients, your staff, and your doctor. Most of the suffering in relationships comes from the futile hope of getting the other person to change.

FIGURE 5: The spectrum of the new patient experience.

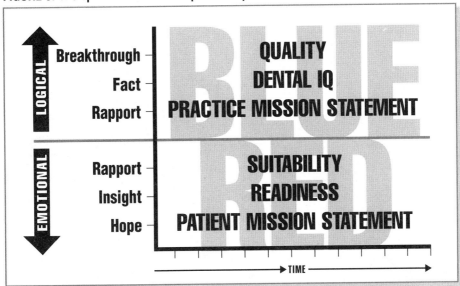

Dr. Brian Spillman paraphrases a popular axiom, *"If we want to influence our patients' perspective, don't ask them to look further than they can see."*

Instead of investing your energy into making patients ready by raising their dental IQ, use your energy to identify and serve those who are ready.

Would you rather have patients with high dental IQ or patients who are ready?

CHAPTER 11

If You
BUILD IT,
Will They
Come?

The Structure of
Selling Complete Dentistry

In the process of selling complete dentistry the structure is the sequence and content of appointments, which shape the relationship with the patient, that ultimately leads to case acceptance. The structure of selling complete dentistry and creating relationships is like whistling: it's easier to do than it is to explain. Building the right structure of your case acceptance process makes it easier to create relationships. And if you build it, they will come.

In my previous book, *Dentists: An Endangered Species*, I named the structure of selling complete dentistry the "No-Contest Case Presentation." I wrote the book in 1996 and in the years since I have enjoyed hearing about the collective experience of several hundred dentists who have successfully implemented part or all of the No-Contest structure. To get the most out of the following chapters on the structure of selling complete dentistry, I strongly recommend you read or read again *Dentists: An Endangered Species* (see www.paulhomoly.com for information about the book). As you will see, it contains information essential for obtaining the greatest benefits from this book.

The Six Steps

In chapter 2, I introduced the concept of structure. Again, there are six steps in the structure of selling complete dentistry:

1. Initial experience
2. Diagnostic appointment
3. Case preview
4. Case discussion
5. Case discussion letter
6. Preoperative appointment

These six steps assume that one dentist is doing all aspects of care. In the team approach to care, in which general dentists work with other general dentists or specialists, seven steps exist in the structure of selling complete dentistry. I've indicated in which office each step is completed.

They are:
1. Initial experience—GP
2. Diagnostic appointment—GP
3. Case preview—GP
4. Case discussion—GP
5. Referral—Specialist
6. Case discussion letter—GP and specialist
7. Preoperative appointment—GP and specialist

Just because there are six or seven steps in the structure doesn't mean there are six or seven appointments. You'll learn later, or you may already know from *Dentists: An Endangered Species*, that the entire structure can be completed in as few as two appointments.

The Five Critical Dialogues

Five critical dialogues are woven into the whole structure. Over the years, I've learned that mastering these five critical dialogues is the weakest link in the process of implementing this case acceptance process. It is difficult for many people because mastering these dialogues demands that you use the information in the chapters on philosophy and the communication skills.

I've labeled the critical dialogues CD-1, CD-2, and so forth. They are:

CD-1: Identifying and appointing the compelled target patient.

CD-2: Choosing between the lifetime strategy versus chief complaint.

CD-3: Introducing the concept of dental budget.

CD-4: Previewing the treatment plan in the future tense—case preview.

CD-5: Determining the budget.

This chapter provides an overview of each critical dialogue, thereby giving you a sense of the content and the sequence of the entire structure. Then in succeeding chapters greater detail is given about each step and its accompanying critical dialogue.

Critical Dialogue Number One (CD-1)

CD-1 is about identifying and appointing the compelled target patient. This dialogue takes place over the telephone between the new patient and the scheduler. The responsibility of the scheduler is to appoint the compelled target patient into the schedule so the clinical team has time to create a positive initial experience.

Critical Dialogue Number Two (CD-2)

CD-2 occurs at a first appointment immediately after a simple initial examination is completed. In CD-2 the dentist asks: *"Are you more interested in just having your chief complaint (black tooth, sore spot, and so forth) fixed, or are you more interested in pursuing a lifetime strategy of dental health? What's best for you now?"* This question guides us to the most appropriate care for this patient, demonstrates that we're willing to provide great service, and reduces our frustration and wasted time by eliminating the long complete dentistry examination and consultation on people who aren't interested or aren't ready.

Critical Dialogue Number Three (CD-3)

CD-3 introduces the concept of the dental budget to those patients who have elected to pursue a lifetime strategy of dental health. This dialogue between the dentist and the patient is in the form of a question: *"I'm really good about staying within a budget if I know I need to. Have you thought about your budget at all?"*

This dialogue is not intended to help you learn a patient's budget but rather foreshadows a future definitive discussion about realistic budgets and the appropriate dentistry that fits the person's budget. The number one concern most patients have about complete care is its cost. CD-3 assures them you'll provide care within their budget.

Critical Dialogue Number Four (CD-4)

CD-4 is delivered by the dentist and is structured in *future* tense. It is designed to inform the patient of what's possible but stops short of carving that recommendation in stone.

For example, during CD-4 you may say: *"A good way to make your front teeth beautiful is to fuse a thin, enamel-colored coating over them. They're called laminate veneers and when you're ready, and it fits within your budget, that would be a good way to go."* CD-4 hints at treatment recommendations and gives patients hope.

Critical Dialogue Number Five (CD-5)

CD-5 determines the patient's dental budget and occurs after the patient has an idea of what's possible but is not fully aware of its cost. CD-5 is in the form of a reminder from the dentist:

"Last time, I recommended that you think about your dental budget. Give me an idea what you're comfortable with and I guarantee you I'll design your care to fit within that budget." CD-5 opens the dialogue of balancing your dentistry with the patient's budget. The dentistry that doesn't fall within the budget is planned for succeeding years. The goal is to not dilute the quality or comprehensiveness of treatment, but to implement the best plan over time.

Over the next several chapters, I'll discuss in detail the six/ seven step structure of case acceptance for complete dentistry and show you how the five critical dialogues fit within them.

CHAPTER 12

Just Who
DO YOU THINK
You're Talking To?

Identifying and Appointing
the Target Patient

Wouldn't it be wonderful if you knew that your new patient caller is a compelled target patient, ready for complete care? If you did, would you squeeze the patient's initial visit in between two screaming kids, or would you reserve a quiet, sane spot in your schedule? This chapter is about creating the time and space to start off on the right foot with complete care patients.

The structure of case acceptance for complete dentistry starts with Critical Dialogue Number One (CD-1), which identifies and appoints the compelled target patient. This dialogue takes place over the telephone between the new patient and the scheduler.

It's been my experience and the experience of many of my clients that new patient procedures can be effectively grouped on Monday afternoons and Tuesday mornings. I like early-in-the-week appointments for new patients because they're not yet dealing with the hassles of the entire week, so they still have the energy and the right attitude to make health care decisions. Of course, the same is true for you and your staff. You are all more chipper early in the week. In the dental office, I don't think anything good happens after Wednesdays.

My staff and I generally booked two new patients every hour. Because I had two consultation areas it was easy for my two assistants and I to see six new patients in a three-hour period. Because we didn't have any time-consuming procedures during this time, we enjoyed total flexibility in managing each new patient.

Most dentists block out hours in their schedule for production and have specific times of the day and days of the week they prefer to reserve for these appointments. I recommend that you also block hours for communication appointments, new patient examinations, and consultations, for which CD-2 through CD-5 are designed.

When you meet consecutive new patients and are not burdened with running back into an operatory to make an impression, your personal skills are sharper, you stay on time more easily, and you'll demonstrate a better attitude because you're less stressed.

Blocking in appointment time for new patients and consultations reduces the stress of shifting from a blue spectrum activity (fixing a tooth) to red spectrum (new patient communications).

Dr. Tom Kellog from Howell, Michigan offers his perspective on scheduling:

"Our whole team loves doing examinations/consultations batched together. We see our new patients on Mondays twice a month. Our energy level is much higher because it's early in the workweek and our minds aren't wandering, perhaps thinking about a restorative procedure going on in another room. It's difficult to go from one room where I'm doing a restorative procedure to an examination, a time my mind should be focused on building a relationship. Batching examinations has eliminated this problem. Our new patients see us as more organized and they can see that we have structured time for them and we have our 'act' together.

"My staff also thinks batching examinations is great. Before we restructured examination times, we'd see these appointments almost as if they were emergencies, tucked in-between production. That was stressful to everyone. Now the stress is gone."

Critical Dialogue Number One (CD-1)

During the compelled patient initial appointment, be prepared to do a variety of things ranging from a complete examination, an extraction, partial denture repair, a bite adjustment, and so forth. Flexibility in the new patient process allows you to do any of these procedures, stay on time, and make the patient happy—without any added stress!

Some patients do not reveal themselves as compelled, but a few questions over the telephone can bring them out of the closet. Most adult compelled patients are missing many teeth, so asking "Are you wearing full or partial dentures or have you been advised to wear them?" will launch the conversation about missing teeth.

When identifying compelled patients consider the distance the patient drives to your office. "How long will it take you to drive here?" or "How far away are you?" are questions that give you an idea about how many other offices the new patient is driving by to get to yours. If the patient is traveling more than an hour to see you, that person is compelled.

Age is another indicator of being compelled. Older patients are usually more compelled than younger patients. Ask for date of birth during CD-1 to gracefully discover the patient's age. Individuals over fifty are good candidates for being compelled patients.

Most practices would sell more dentistry if the patient base were twenty years older.

Since older patients are more likely to be compelled, many practices struggle with selling complete dentistry because they have too many young patients in their practice. You'll suffer when you try to talk a thirty-year-old into a posterior three-unit bridge.

If you have focused on providing procedures for younger patients, i.e., air abrasion, pedodontics, cosmetic care, sealants, orthodontics, chances are your patient base has few real candidates for rehabilitative complete care. Imagine yourself in the car repair business. Would you do more business with new cars or old cars? Old cars are good for business, as are older patients.

If during CD-1 your patient reveals he is from out of town, has many missing teeth, hates the way he looks and chews, is fifty years old, and is anxious to get an appointment, be prepared to "take yes for an answer." It's your job to remove any obstacles from his path to complete care. Those obstacles include: the time you make the patient wait before he or she can see you, mandatory complete examinations, multiple hygiene visits, and most patient education efforts. Your goal is to put target patients in the right places at the right times, but you can't do this unless you identify them on the telephone.

StorySelling and CD-1

Abundant opportunities exist to use StorySelling during CD-1. Tell stories about people who share your caller's location, chief complaint and concerns, or medical and dental history. YourStory is a good one to tell if you have a scared or hesitant caller. Remember, these stories are short—fifteen seconds max! When you're speaking on the telephone you lose the impact of body language and facial expression and have to rely on tone of voice and the meaning of your words. You need some attitude when storytelling on the telephone or else you'll put people to sleep.

Do you know whom you're talking to? Find out by identifying and appointing the compelled target patient.

CHAPTER 13

If **YOGI BERRA** Had Been a Dentist

The New Patient's Initial Experience

If Yogi Berra had been a dentist he would have said: "Ninety percent of the patient's initial experience is mental, the other half is clinical." Does this sound confusing? It's not half as confusing as most of us sound to our patients when we overwhelm them with technical details at their initial visit. If you want them to play ball with you, then the new patient experience for complete care patients needs to be more mental than clinical.

Assuming you've identified and appointed target patients (CD-1), the next step is to get them in and start the new patient interview. I often hear this question during my seminars: "Who should conduct the new patient interview, a staff member or the doctor?"

Put yourself in the patient's place. Who would you rather talk to, a staff member or the doctor? New patients are in your office for one reason, and that's to see the doctor. I don't mean to slight the many high-energy staff members, who may also be good communicators, but patients deserve the opportunity to go to the head of the line.

I know it's more efficient to have a staff person review medical and dental history, interview patients, and report her findings to the doctor. But is it more effective? Poll your patients at their recall appointments on who they would prefer to talk with during the new patient interview. You'll find that most complete dentistry target patients prefer to talk with the doctor.

"But what if our doctor is not a good communicator?" some staff members complain. "Wouldn't it be better to have a strong communicator to make a great first impression?" I agree with that solution, but for the short term only. If you're a weak communicator and rely on staff people to build relationships for you, you never will reach the level that's possible if you build your own communication skills.

For most dentists, building stronger communication skills provides the greatest leverage for selling complete dentistry.

Seat the new patient in a confidential talking area. Open bay operatories are fine for kids but are the worse possible environment to discuss emotionally charged issues with new patients. Do what it takes to create a confidential area.

The dentist starts the new patient interview with a simple question *"How can I help you today?"* Focus immediately on the patient. Resist reciting your mission statement or any statements that center on the office, the doctor, or the staff. After you ask the question, don't interrupt. Stay connected, and resist offering treatment recommendations. Listen to the patient's story and discover how you can build rapport with the patient through storytelling (Chapter 6).

The Simple Examination

After you've listened to the patient's story and have told yours, describe the process of a simple examination. "Casey, let me do a good examination for you. Suzette, my assistant, will take one simple x-ray. After that I'll examine you, and then we'll come back here to talk about things. Is that all right with you?"

Understand the Nature of the Disability

A simple initial examination is a short, overview process in which you gain just enough clinical information to understand the patient's disability, defined as why she is unhappy with her teeth. For example, the patient's chief complaint is that she hates the way her teeth look. During your simple examination you notice black fillings in her front teeth and many missing back teeth. Do you need any more clinical information than that to understand why she hates her teeth? Or a patient tells you he can't eat and during the simple examination, you discover that his full dentures move one-half inch when he speaks and the radiograph of his mandible reveals a bone height of 10 mm. Do you need any more clinical information to understand why this patient has trouble chewing?

For most patients the simple examination takes ten minutes and most also have a relatively obvious disability: ugly teeth, can't chew, infection, and so forth. Patients usually talk about their disabilities in simple ways: "I hate the way I look!" This is a patient-centered issue and statement. On the other hand, a diagnosis is dentist centered: severe attrition to the maxillary anterior teeth with an accompanying reverse smile line. Determining the diagnosis and treatment plan requires a complete, not simple, examination.

Don't confuse understanding the patient's disability (red spectrum) with diagnosis and treatment planning (blue spectrum).

A simple examination consists of an oral cancer screening examination, a periodontal screening examination, a panoral radiograph, a simple tooth charting, and a medical and dental history. You can do a simple examination in ten minutes. The goal of the simple examination is to move through the clinical aspect of the new patient experience and return to the communication aspect.

You sell complete dentistry by being a great communicator, not by overwhelming patients with diagnostic procedures they don't understand or may not want.

If you don't have the capacity to make panoral radiographs, you're significantly handicapped during the simple examination process. Full- mouth intraoral radiographs usually aren't needed to understand the basis of the patient's disability. They're time and labor intensive, patients hate and fear them, and they are poor visual aids. Save the intraoral radiograph ordeal until after the patient has decided to consider a lifetime strategy for dental health.

After the simple examination you still might not understand the basis of the patient's disability. For example, the chief complaint may be: "Oh, doctor, whenever I eat strawberries pain starts in my scalp and runs down the backs of my legs." You look into the person's mouth and see thirty-two perfect teeth. Chances are you will never understand why this patient is unhappy.

If you cannot reasonably understand the basis of the patient's disability, chances are excellent that this is a patient you shouldn't treat. Patients like this are good candidates for referral to a colleague who can understand her situation—or for referral to a dentist you hate!

Prove Yourself

If you see an obvious problem related to aesthetics, phonetics, infection, or pain it's good dentistry, and good business, too, to take care of the immediate problem first. There are two examinations going on: yours and the patient's. To pass the patient's examination and prove yourself, taking care of an immediate problem is a great way to build trust.

It always makes good sense to let patients experience your care, your touch, and your attitude before you ask them to make major decisions about their dental health.

Dr. Mark Davis of Clearwater, Florida believes it's important to prove yourself to patients. When Mark senses the patient needs assurance or if he sees an obvious disability that is easily remedied, Mark fixes the problem before he asks if the patient is interested in complete care. Here's his sample dialogue: *"'Karen, let me show you what I can do and what it's like to experience treatment in this office. This will give you a better understanding of what I can do for you.' After I've helped them, most people arrange to be treated as quickly as they can."*

Make the Patient Right

After the simple examination and/or providing simple care to relieve an acute problem, the patient returns to the consultation area, where we will accomplish three things:

1. **Make the patient right.**
2. **Give the patient hope.**
3. **Offer the patient a choice.**

This structure is repeated during many conversations with both new and established patients in various situations, including: following examinations, conversations initiated after consultations, and during telephone conversations. Throughout this book I present the structure, the critical dialogues, and then suggest words that work within the structure.

> **Don't try to memorize words; understand structure and the words will naturally come.**

Make the Patient Right

Make the patient right by confirming that you understand why she feels the way she does about her teeth. "Mrs. Salsbury, I can see why you're disappointed with the appearance of your teeth," or "Ms. Crawford, I sure can understand why you have trouble eating. Your dentures don't work very well and I'm surprised you do as well as you do." Resist getting into solutions, recommendations, reprimands, or mission statements. This experience is about the patient, not you.

Making people right embodies a calming and supportive attitude. Let patients know you understand why they're unhappy with their teeth. Telling them how to fix them, which puts you in the blue spectrum, isn't as powerful at this point as empathizing with their situation, which keeps you in the red spectrum.

Give the Patient Hope

Next, give patients hope. Let them know they've come to the right place and you've treated hundreds of patients just like them. "Andy, I've treated hundreds of cases like yours. I know you're discouraged about your teeth. I've helped many people just like you."

Be careful not to recommend treatment at this point. Making them aware that their situation can be helped is much more powerful than launching into a show-and-tell about crowns and veneers.

Offer Your Patients a Choice: CD-2

After you've made patients right and given them hope, offer a choice. The choice is CD-2. The choice is between treating only their chief complaint or developing a lifetime strategy of dental health. You've made this choice easier by relieving any acute problem such as broken front teeth, cracked fillings, painful teeth, and so on.

In CD-2 the dentist asks the key question: *"Are you more interested in just having your chief complaint (whatever that is, i.e., black tooth, sore spot, etc.,) fixed, or are you interested in pursuing a lifetime strategy of dental health. What's best for you now?"*

This question guides us to the most suitable care for this patient, demonstrates our willingness to provide great service, and reduces our frustration and wasted time by eliminating the long, complete dentistry examination and consultation for people who aren't interested or aren't ready.

The tough part about asking this question is in accepting the answer. It's frustrating when a patient with a mouth full of problems opts for fixing the black front tooth only. The biggest mistake I've made during the new patient experience is being judgmental about people with nasty teeth who didn't care. My judgmental attitude came out in my voice and body language, and patients knew I didn't respect or appreciate them.

I'm sure I chased away a practice full of patients because they didn't see their dental health the way I wanted them to see it.

There's a fine line here. The line is between letting people know what's good for them and not being pushy and judgmental. I learned a critical lesson: *The patient who has a mouth full of problems and is only interested in the chief complaint is not wrong, she is just not ready.* When I lightened up and let people pursue things on their own timetable, I eventually did rehabilitation work on folks who, years earlier, let me treat their chief complaint only.

The question within CD-2: *"Are you more interested in just having your chief complaint (i.e., black tooth, sore spot, etc.,) fixed, or are you more interested in pursuing a lifetime strategy of dental health. What's best for you now?"* provides a clear and simple path for you and the patients to follow.

Some of my clients prefer a less formal approach to CD-2. Their dialogue sounds like this. *"Are you more interested in just having your chief complaint (i.e., black tooth, sore spot, etc.,) fixed, or are you interested in having all your teeth fixed. What's best for you now?"* Use the words you're comfortable with.

Dr. Sheldon Hough of Yucca Valley, California talks about CD-2. *"I feel so much more comfortable now in case presentation and I know my patients are, too. I have a bread-and-butter practice in a medium sized town and I have to be careful not to blow people out of the water quoting big fees. By letting people know that it's possible to pursue a lifetime strategy for dental health over a period of time, it puts people at ease and let's them know that I care. In the past I've tried to communicate that I care, but I've never had the words. The phrase "lifetime strategy" communicates I care and it takes down the barriers almost immediately."*

Treating the patient's chief complaint is part of the examination a patient does on you.

Most new patients (90 percent) in a general practice will choose to have their chief complaint treated. Cheerfully accept their choice and treat the complaint as soon as possible. You may have already started relieving their problem at the beginning of the appointment. As you evolve into seeing your new patients and consults on Monday afternoons or Tuesday mornings, you have the time and rooms to fix the chief complaint.

If your patient has a nagging problem and you fix it fast, painlessly—and without whining—you've passed his examination. If you don't have the time to treat this patient, reschedule him ASAP. It's especially important that you know if your patient is from out of town, information you gather in CD-1. Give yourself time to fix the chief complaint so this patient won't have to make the return trip.

After the chief complaint is relieved, restate your offer to develop a lifetime strategy. If he still isn't ready, put him on recall and ask for referrals. At every recall appointment, the hygienist should remind him of the lifetime strategy option.

If the patient opts for a lifetime strategy for dental health, put the patient right back into the operatory, and perform a *complete* examination, which is the diagnostic appointment.

Dr. Joe Shae, a prosthodontist in St. Louis, Illinois, talks about the importance of not pushing patients past their chief complaints.

"The number one thing that I've learned is not to challenge people. To some extent they're either ready or not ready. I think dentists create a problem by trying to make patients ready when they're clearly not. There are people in dentistry teaching dentists how to use fancy closing questions to get people who aren't ready to say yes. But this sets up a challenge somewhere along the line. Even if they say yes today, then they may be the ones who won't show up for their next appointment or they'll become slow-pay patients. Philosophically, just this concept of doing what patients want when they're ready has been great.

"We've always done the chief complaint first to some extent. Yesterday we saw a new patient, John Powers, who needed new dentures. They're twenty years old and nasty—he has sore spots all over his mouth and a big nasty spot on the lower front in areas #21-23. He was a patient of a dentist of about an hour south of here. This dentist is a young associate in the practice. The associate looked at John and said, 'You need new dentures.' The associate wouldn't touch him and said, 'You need new dentures' and didn't adjust the denture to relieve the soreness. John left the office and called us. We scheduled him as a new patient and blocked out an hour for his appointment. We took

him back in the operatory and my assistant came up to me and told me that John just wanted his denture adjusted. 'Don't give him the whole dog-and-pony show. He just wants the adjustment,' she said. I went in and asked John how he was doing.

"John said 'Oh, I got this spot. Can you fix it?'

"'Be glad to fix it.' I used a little pressure indicating paste and shaved off and overextended flange...John loved it. No lectures or opinions. We gave him just what he wanted. He was almost in tears as he shook my hand.

"'That's great!' John said. 'You know, I'd like to have you make me a new set of dentures.'"

Nordstrom's or the Ritz Carlton is Not for Everyone

I want to be very clear about this point: *Don't feel obligated to put all patients through the CD-2 process. Focus CD-2 on target patients.* If your target patient is an older adult who needs rehabilitative dentistry, CD-2 makes sense. For the young adult who needs a few fillings, an examination, and cleaning, CD-2 might be overkill. Get nontarget patients in and out: "Treat 'em and street 'em," or in other words, treat them great, and they'll love you for it.

I've heard and read some interesting comparisons related to customer service between dental offices and high-end hotels and department stores such as Ritz Carlton, Nordstrom, and so on. I agree that we should emulate the spirit of customer service that these great businesses demonstrate. But it concerns me when attempts at customer service go too far. Here's a summary of a telephone conversation I've had more than once:

"Hello, Dr. Homoly, I'm Dr. Joe Blow and I want you to help me change my practice."

"Great. Tell me about your practice and what you'd like to do," I say.

"I want to knock my patients' socks off with outstanding service. I want them to come to my office ready, willing, and able. I want them to have the experience of their life. I want a practice like a Nordstrom store, or Ritz Carlton, where the staff will go to great lengths to make customers happy. Extraordinary one-of-a-kind service that makes people run out and tell their friends about us! Can you help me?"

"No, I can't," I reply.

An awkward pause follows.

"Nobody can make people run into a dental office expecting the time of their life. People don't go to dental offices for fun experiences. They go on vacation for that. The best I can do is to help you give your patients a pleasantly memorable experience that surpasses their expectations. Will they run out and tell all their friends? Probably not. People are too occupied with their own lives to go too far out of their way to make you happy. I've been in dentistry for twenty-five years and I've never met a dentist who has filled his practice with patients who are ready, willing, and able who were referred from previous patients."

Attempting to overserve, oversell, or build relationships with people who aren't interested sounds and feels like selling—manipulation—to patients.

I hate bursting bubbles, but worse than that, I hate going into an office that has unrealistic expectations. If Nordstrom and the Ritz Carlton have cracked the universal code of customer service and appeal for dentistry, then why aren't they operating dental offices?

Let's stay real.

Not every new patient is looking for or needs lifelong relationships with their dentist. Many of them want you to fix their tooth and get on their way. Rolling the red carpet out for them just slows them down. You and your staff don't want to attempt to build meaningful relationships or experience deep empathy with every patient. You'll burn out. *Get 'em in, get 'em out, and make 'em happy.* Happy patients return when they're ready to get their teeth fixed.

One of my dentist clients put himself and his staff through sales training, and one of his hygienists told me an interesting story. "We were taught these scripted responses that all the staff hated," she said. "When a patient would complain about the expense of a procedure, we were supposed to say, 'Think of the fee for dentistry as an investment in your dental health.' I had one patient laugh in my face and ask me if I had just taken a sales course." Ouch! Assume your patients are sophisticated and can spot a canned response when they hear one.

Positive Framing

It's important that complete care patients know what's good about their mouths. If you have bad teeth, you've heard the same bad news in every dentist's office you've been in. We've been trained to find defects and inform patients about them. We have not been trained in ways to talk to patients about the positive features of their mouths. Dr. James Pride calls this "positive framing."

Do you know how refreshing it is for a dental cripple to hear what's good about him?

I've always had weak eyes. I've had six eye surgeries and have worn glasses or contact lenses all my life. I also am red-green color-blind. The only tests I'd ever flunk are the ones I took in the optometrist's office. I am very tired about hearing bad news about my eyes.

In March of 2000, I was evaluated for Lasik laser eye surgery. Dr. Jonathan Christenbury is my surgeon. He finished his examination and said: "You've got great eyes for this procedure. The health of your eyes is good, your correction is within the range of this surgery, you have adequate tear flow, and your ocular pressure is fine." He went on about all the good things about my eyes that indicated me as a candidate for this surgery. Yes, I know he is in the business of eye surgery, but it felt great to hear someone say nice things about my eyes.

Tell patients what is good about their mouths. I don't care if she has class three mobility, severe end-stage periodontal disease, occlusal disease, and bad breath, for every defect I can find, I guarantee you I can find a good thing.

Here's a sample dialogue of positive framing with a patient with end-stage dental disease. Her chief complaint is a broken lateral incisor. I've just completed a simple examination. I'm going to make the patient right, give her hope, and offer her a choice. And I'm going to accomplish this using positive framing.

"Colleen, I understand why you're disappointed in the appearance and comfort of your teeth. I see how the missing and loose teeth can make you feel self-conscious of your mouth. You and I both know that you have some severe problems with your teeth. I treat many folks just like you and what they often don't realize is all the good things about their teeth. In your case, Colleen, you have some very good things going for you. Your bone structure beneath your teeth is excellent. The bottom border of your lower jaw is well shaped and formed. The relationship between your upper and lower jaw is excellent. I know a lot of patients who would love to have the remaining healthy bone you have. Your sinuses look healthy, your saliva flow is excellent, and the overall health of the gums not associated with the teeth is great. Yes, you have problems with the part of your mouth that you can see, but underneath it all, things look good.

"But before we decide what to do for you, let me ask you, are you interested in fixing the front tooth, or are you interested in talking about how we can fix all your teeth? What's best for you now?"

The Spectrum of Appeal

Let's put CD-2 on the Spectrum of Appeal. (See figure 1.) Diagnosis and treatment planning are blue spectrum activities. They are what we want and like to do. They are *quality* issues.

FIGURE 1: The initial experience.

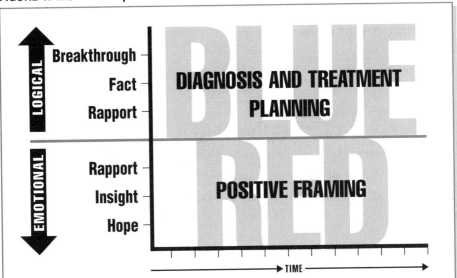

On the other hand, positive framing is a red spectrum event to patients and is a *suitability* issue. It makes them feel good about themselves and us. To sell complete dentistry you need both spectra. What most of my clients miss is the red spectrum because they are focused on the thoroughness of the examination and discussing treatment options.

Let's make a distinction between health and hope. There is a strong blue spectrum component to health: freedom from pain and infection, adequate zones of attached gingiva, anterior guidance that discludes posterior teeth in eccentric movements, and so forth. However, hope is completely red spectrum. Which is easier for the patient to understand and experience, health or hope? I'd vote for hope every time. Total focus on health issues during patients' initial experience with us disconnects them from us.

When you discuss health issues, always include hope issues. Blend logical and emotional appeal.

Unstructured Selling Opportunities

Unstructured selling opportunities occur when the boss isn't around, and an employee gives you straight-from-the-hip advice on what's *really* going on in the business. For example, you're in a restaurant and you ask your waitress, "How's the salmon today?"

She says, "It's okay, but if you'd like fish today, I'd try the red snapper. A lot of my customers tell me they like the snapper better than the salmon."

Now, let's say you ask the same question of the chef. "Hey, Frenchie, how's the salmon today?" Is he likely to give you his opinion or his customers' opinion? His own, of course. And whose opinion are you more apt to be persuaded by, the waitress' or the chef's? I go with the waitress' every time because she's the one who gets the looks from her customers and has to go toe-to-toe with people who don't like the food. The waitress is in an unstructured selling opportunity. She may not be an expert, but she knows what her customers like.

Structured selling opportunities occur when the boss or someone with an obvious vested interest (such as the chef) tells you what to think and do. In the dental office, the case presentation and most conversations with the doctor or office manager or financial coordination are structured selling opportunities. In the dental office, the staff is the waitresses and the doctor is the chef.

Unstructured selling opportunities constantly occur for the dental assistant in the new patient process. She may not be an expert, but she knows what her customers like.

Let's say your dental assistant is aligning the patient in the panoral machine and the patient asks, "What does this thing do?" Or as your assistant is taking the patient to the operatory he spots a picture of a beautiful smile on the wall and asks, "What is this?" Or you've completed the simple examination and your assistant is bringing the patient up front to the consultation room, and she says, "Your doctor seems young (or old, or quiet, or loud, or in a hurry)." Or you walk out of the operatory, and the patient leans over to the assistant and says, "I'm concerned about money. Is this work very expensive?"

Whatever the staff member says will be a strong indicator of what is really going on in your office. Do you know what your assistants are saying after you leave the room? Most dentists don't. The best way to optimize unstructured selling opportunities is to be aware of them, as well as prepared for them. Too often the assistants are breaking down and setting up rooms, and otherwise hustling around. They don't make opportunities or aren't given the chance to sell in an unstructured way. In the next chapter I discuss an unstructured selling opportunity called the "Golden Moment." It might be the most influential communication during new patient experiences.

StorySelling and CD-2

Remember that CD-2 asks the key question: *"Are you interested in having me treat your chief complaint or put together a lifetime strategy for dental health. What's best for you now?"* In response, patients often ask: *"What's a lifetime strategy for dental health?"* This is also a key question and a good way to answer it combines logic with the *"Lifetime Strategy for Dental HealthStory."*

For example, a response to, "What's a lifetime strategy for dental health?" may sound like this. (Logic, blue spectrum, is printed in **bold**; emotion/story, red spectrum, is printed in *italics*.)

"Bonnie, a lifetime strategy is created when we plan your dentistry to give you the best possible dental health for the rest of your life. Most people have never had one."

"I just finished Florence, who reminds me of you. She had problems with her teeth all her life. When she turned forty, she decided to fix her teeth. We planned her care so she would keep her teeth for the rest of her life. We can do the same for you."

In response to, "What's a lifetime strategy for dental health?" tell the story of other patients who didn't know, had the plan, completed care, and now love their teeth and their life.

Following the simple exam, be prepared to tell the *Making You RightStory* and the *Giving You HopeStory*. And great opportunities for StorySelling are the "Golden Moments." These are the great opportunities to use StorySelling when the patient asks a critical question at a time your staff members least expect it or have time to answer it.

Take the Fork in the Road

CD-2 takes the ambiguity out of the relationship with the patient. Many of my clients have patients who have been in limbo for years, with no one knowing what the next step is, nor its priority. Both you and your patient need to commit to a plan. That plan is either we "fix your teeth as they break," or we put together a plan that will map out total dental health. Any plan that falls between these two is administratively and clinically hard to manage.

CD-2 creates a fork in the road. One way leads to treating the chief complaint, the other to a lifetime strategy. As Yogi Berra would say: "When you come to a fork in the road, take it."

To summarize, figure 2 shows the structural flow of CD-1 and CD-2. CD-1 identifies target-compelled patients on the telephone so they can be appropriately appointed for the new patient experience. Make note of any nagging chief complaint and anticipate fixing it.

During the simple initial examination, determine the basis of the disability. After the examination, make the patient right, give him hope, and offer a choice. The choice is CD-2: Treat the chief complaint or choose a lifetime strategy for dental health, or the alternative phrase, fixing all the teeth. Do all of this in the spirit of positive framing.

If the patient opts to only fix the chief complaint, cheerfully comply, fix it ASAP, and re-offer the lifetime strategy. If he refuses, put him on recall and re-offer the lifetime strategy option at every recall appointment. If he accepts the offer, move on to the complete examination, the diagnostic appointment (See chapter 15.) Either way, you and the patient are still playing ball. Yogi Berra would be proud.

FIGURE 2: The initial experience.

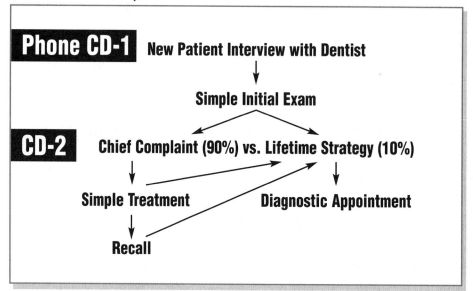

CHAPTER 14

DIAGNOSING
The
Wallet

━━━━━━━━━━━━━━━━━━━━━━━━

The Diagnostic Appointment

If you want to embarrass patients and make them angry, recommend treatment without knowing what they can afford. But if you want to please patients, ask them what they can afford. I can sense you resisting what I'm saying. "No way, Jose," you might tell me. "I can't ask them what they can afford. They'll think I'm diagnosing their wallet."

You already diagnose their wallet. You do it by offering complete care and quoting a big fee. "No," the patient says, "what else can you do?" Then you offer plan B with a lower fee. The patient says, "Still too much." You offer plan C with the lowest fee, and the patient finally says okay. Congratulations, you've just diagnosed that person's wallet. You did it by trial, error, blood, sweat, and tears. It's a lot easier on everyone to ask about budget before you recommend treatment.

The diagnostic appointment occurs after the patient agrees to pursue a lifetime strategy for dental health (CD-2). It may take place during the simple examination. If you've given yourself enough time and flexibility (CD-1), and the patient has indicated he wants comprehensive planning (CD-2), then it's a simple matter of putting him back into the operatory, which has been left set up for him, and completing the full examination.

It's at the diagnostic appointment that you bring out the heavy artillery of your complete examination: study models, face bow, bite registration, complete tooth and periodontal charting, pulp testing, smile analysis, intra oral radiographs, intra oral photographs, TMJ exam, and so on. It makes sense to do the complete examination because the patient wants to develop a lifetime approach to dental health and a complete examination is part of that process.

The Golden Moment

There is a wonderful unstructured selling opportunity immediately following the complete examination, when the doctor leaves the operatory and the assistant is preparing the patient to go up front. I call it the "Golden Moment" because it is an important and unique opportunity to give the patient the right message and advance the selling process. After the doctor leaves the room, patients often ask a question or make a comment to the assistant such as:

"Wow, I had no idea so much goes into this."

"I never had an examination like this before."

"This seems like a lot of work— is this going to be expensive?"

"No offense, but I hate dentists."

"I know I need a lot of work, and has he done many cases like mine," or simply, "I hate needles!"

Ask any dental assistant and she'll tell you patients ask her more pointed and direct questions and reveal their true feelings to her rather than to the doctor.

The questions or comments that occur at the Golden Moment are predictable. The responses should be, too. We know that we're going to hear more or less the same comments/questions about the examination and treatment process.

It's like baseball. Every pitch is a surprise to the batter. But what if just before the pitcher went into his windup, the catcher tapped the batter on the knee and said, "Fastball, low and inside." And sure enough, the pitch is low and inside and the batter rips a double down the left field line. Next time up, the catcher said, "Slow curve, high and outside," and the batter tags one over the second baseman's head.

Baseball is easy when you know what pitch is coming. And in dentistry we know what pitch is coming. Patients are going to ask you the same questions every time: *How much does it cost, How long will it take, How much will it hurt, How much will my insurance pay, and Do I really need all this work?*

No matter how annoying, you're going to be asked the same questions. As Yogi Berra said: "I wish I had an answer to that because I'm tired of answering the question."

Golden Moment Dialogues

The best Golden Moment dialogues are great stories. Become good at telling stories in response to questions/comments about money, treatment time, pain, insurance, and the classic question: *"Do I really need this much dentistry?"*

Here's a typical scenario. You just walked out of the operatory following a conversation with your patient, Sandy, about a cosmetic rehabilitation involving twenty-four teeth. After you're out of earshot, Sandy turns to your assistant Suzette and asks: "Do I really need this much dentistry? He wants to work on all my teeth!"

"It does seem like a lot of work," Suzette says. *"We just finished Becky's cosmetic care. She's a patient of ours who had dark spaces between her front teeth and she hated how she looked when she laughed. Just like you we made every tooth in her smile look great. You'll look great, too."*

Review StorySelling (chapter 6) and get ready for Golden Moments.

Create Golden Moments

Golden Moments create golden opportunities. During their training, make it a point to teach the staff how to handle Golden Moments. Dental assistants should know to *go out of their way* to create Golden Moments. Instead of hustling the patient back up front following the examination, wouldn't it be wonderful if the assistant rolled her stool up to the patient and answered questions and comments in a way that communicated to the patient that she was in the right place to get her teeth fixed. She'll have time to do this if the new patient experience is appointed to allow for flexibility and adequate time (CD-1).

Chair-side dental assistants can be the most influential people in the practice. They spend the most time with the patient, are in a position to do the most unstructured selling, and have the opportunity to build the closest relationships.

The chair-side dental assistant is the person whose communication skills I would invest in most enthusiastically.

Unfortunately, continuing education in dentistry ignores the opportunity to build great communication skills in chair-side dental assistants. The closest most of them come to training in communication skills involves personality profiles or learning to smile into a mirror while talking on the telephone. These skills aren't wrong, but they're woefully incomplete. Most dental assistants come away from the traditional communications skills courses without the ability and confidence to present the most appealing aspects of the practice, tell compelling stories of successful patients, explain why they work in the office, and answer the truly tough and important questions. This book, the companion audio and video program, the web site, and case acceptance coaching workshop are designed to develop professional skills of the most influential, yet unrecognized, member of the dental team, the chair-side dental assistant.

Years ago, my good friend and the leading implantologist, Dr. Carl Misch, carried out an informal research project. Once treatment was completed, we asked our patients to tell us who most influenced their decision to undergo treatment. Over 60 percent said it was the chair-side dental assistant. For over twenty years I've worked with some outstanding chair-side dental assistants: Brenda, Jeanna, Renee, Peggy, Linda, Suzette, Libby, Lisa, Jeannie. They all learned to manage the Golden Moment very well. I'm convinced that they "sold" our patients on comprehensive care, and I confirmed the sale during the case presentation process.

The Diagnostic Review

After the complete examination and Golden Moments comes the diagnostic review. This conversation with patients centers on the value of the examination. Return them to the confidential talking area. Remember the structure of the conversation: *make them right, give them hope, give them a choice.* Then "Play it again, Sam." Make your patients right by giving a short overview of your findings, emphasizing the things you see that are good about their dental health, which, as you recall, is positive framing. Full rehabilitative candidates often know what's wrong with them, but are unaware or do not fully appreciate what is right. Make them right. Give them hope by telling them they can be helped or offer a story about a patient just like them whom you helped. Then give them a choice. And don't forget to ask what questions or comments they have.

Here's a sample diagnostic review conversation:

"Mrs. Bamber, I see a lot of good things about your mouth. The underlying bone of your upper and lower jaw is very good. This means you have a strong and solid foundation to support your new teeth. Your sinuses appear to be clear and healthy. Your bite, or the relationship between your upper and lower jaw, is good. This will help us get a predictable result for you. I did an oral cancer screening examination for your today and I find no evidence of cancer. In your age group, 5 percent of all cancers occur in the mouth."

"I know you're disappointed with the appearance of your teeth and you want to chew better. You remind me of Barb, a patient who had similar problems. Her work has been complete for over a year now and she loves her new teeth. You will love your work, too.

"The reason it was important to do the complete examination with all the models and photographs is so I can study your case when you're not here. Next time, after I've had a chance to study your case, we'll talk about how we can help you and by that time, I'll know your case by heart. You've made a good decision to plan your dental care. What questions or comments do you have for me?"

Be careful at this point; do not get into too much detail. Give an overview and focus not on the techniques or processes, but on the planning. Your answers to the comments and questions that follow should be addressed from the perspective that the best answers will be available after you've had a chance to study the case. This technique is called a deferral and is discussed in chapter 4.

Most patients who have chosen to have a lifetime strategy for dental health are usually satisfied to postpone a conversation about specific treatment recommendations and fees.

Critical Dialogue Number Three (CD-3)

Critical Dialogue Number Three (CD-3) introduces the concept of the dental budget. CD-3 occurs just as you're leaving the consultation area. You're about to head to the front desk to book the next appointment. But just as you're ready to move, you say: *"Oh, by the way. I'm really good about staying within a budget if I know I need to. Have you thought about your budget at all?"*

This question is delivered as an aside, a casual comment, as if you just thought of it and remembered it is something important you want the patient to think about. The answer we're looking for is: "No, doc, I haven't, but I'll think about it." *Don't* get heavy and serious and deliver CD-3 as a statement—"Think about your dental budget"—rather than a question. Nor do you ask: "What's your budget?" You want the emphasis to be on the word "thought."

CD-3 is at the heart of selling complete dentistry and adds an entirely new dimension to the doctor-patient relationship. In most traditional case presentation techniques, the fee is disclosed only *after* you've explained the treatment. The treatment plan is presented without regard to the affordability—read "suitability"—of the care. Then after the patient learns the fee, the dentist and patient begin to determine the dentistry that the patient cannot afford at that time. This process devalues the relationship and is uncomfortable for patients, staff, and doctor. Ultimately, the dentist and patient will arrive at the treatment plan that will fit the patient's budget. By using CD-3, you'll present only that part of the lifetime strategy that fits the patient's budget.

Dr. Timothy Droege comments on the concept of dental budget. *"The budget concept is so fundamental. It's like everything else we purchase in our lives. Why in dentistry that never occurred to us is amazing. Using the budget strategy is key to our success."*

The concept of budget includes a patient's time, because some dental patients have more money than time. Many of my clients include questions about the patient's schedule during CD-3: *"Have you thought at all about your budget and schedule?"* After you ask the question, tell the patient that at the next appointment you'll discuss the budget and schedule and decide on a treatment plan that will fit both.

Here's a sample CD-3 dialogue that follows the diagnostic review. It's clear the conversation is over and you're ready to set the next appointment. You're about to leave when you say: *"Oh, by the way. I'm really good about staying within a budget if I know I need to. Have you thought at all about your budget?"*

Here are typical responses:

"Budget for dental care? No I haven't thought of it. I figure you'll tell me what I'll need and I'll tell you whether I can afford it."

"No I haven't. Is it expensive?"

"I'd like to see what my insurance will pay and go from there."

Your responses might be:

"I understand. Most patients don't have a budget for their dentistry. But think about it, and next time we'll discuss how your dental care can best fit within your budget and schedule."

"Dental care can be expensive, but I guarantee you that we will prescribe only the treatment that will comfortably fit within your budget."

"I understand you're interested in using your insurance—most patients are. Next time we'll talk about your care, see how much your insurance will pay, and I guarantee you any treatment we decide on will fit with your budget."

Immediately after your response, end your conversation about budget, and bring the patient to the front desk or wherever you make the next appointments: *"Come with me, Mrs. Lucas. Let's bring you up front and Ginger can help us get your next appointment."* Notice that I didn't start a contest with the patient over her responses. I didn't argue about insurance, make any discouraging comments, or delve into specific fees.

I want my patient to know that I will treat him within his budget. Rarely will a patient say, "Yes I have thought about my budget. It is X dollars." Most of the time you'll catch the patient by surprise with the question because in dental offices no one has ever asked that question.

Traditionally in case presentations, fees are only discussed *after* the treatment plan is explained. It's as if we want patients to want dental care, so we parade it in front of them, but then we must snatch it away when they object to the fee. It's no wonder most doctors hate talking about money. They fear that their good natured show-and-tell case presentation will grind to a halt, and degrade into a negotiation over body-part replacements. Who in their right mind would enjoy this?

Let's Go to Disneyland

Offering patients complete dentistry, but then taking it away because of their budget limitations is a major disappointment for the people we want to work with and help. It's like telling your kids that you're all going to Disneyland, which of course leads to squeals of delight. You add to their enthusiasm by showing them videotapes and brochures of Disneyland. You encourage them to talk to other kids who've been to Disneyland. You show them what they need to know and bring, you assure them that you know how to get there, and you punctuate the whole conversation by telling them that this is going to be the best possible vacation for them—a vacation of a lifetime!

Two weeks before the trip, you call the kids into your den and tell them about the large fees involved in going to Disneyland. First they're surprised, then tears well up in their big eyes.

"We had no idea it was that expensive. We can't afford it."

"No problem. Instead of going to Disneyland, we'll go to Cleveland."

Tell me, how happy are your kids about going to Cleveland? How happy are your patients when they discover they can't afford the care of a lifetime (Disneyland) and you offer to take them to Cleveland? If the budget is not adequate, don't build up their hopes only to dash them later. We want patients to know that Disneyland is a possibility, that you know how to get there, you've been there before, and you'll take them only when it fits within their budget and schedule. (More on our trip to Disneyland in the next chapter.)

Reverse Traditional Thinking

Hundreds of my clients have learned that when the doctor discusses budget issues, it has an amazing way of easing the patient's fee fear. CD-3 foreshadows the conversation you'll have at the next appointment, at which point you will get into specific fees. CD-3 alerts patients that we'll be determining their budget *next time*. I want them to expect it so they're not shocked that all of a sudden I'm talking about money.

Dr. Julie Howard of Savannah, Georgia is three years out of dental school. She says:

Of all the concepts I discuss relative to case acceptance, more dentists appreciate the concept of discussing the budget before offering care more than any other element.

"We all have been excited and so pleased with how we feel about communicating to the patient on a different level—one that helps patients feel good about what they need and allows us to enjoy nurturing our patients at the same time. Recently, my assistant and I had two consultations. Both were successful, but they touched us, too. Because we were so willing to work within their budget, and the patients knew it was okay that we would phase out treatment at their pace, one patient actually broke down in tears of happiness. That was a great feeling! It's wonderful not to struggle with money problems anymore."

Dr. Howard's administrative assistant Johnny says, *"It makes a difference when you say it from the heart. I think the patient knows it. I sit in on the case presentations. The difference in Dr. Julie is unbelievable. She's very confident and she gets to the point. In February of this year Dr. Julie's case acceptance rate was about 68 percent. It is now up to 86 percent acceptance. She's much more poised, she's in control, but she still shows a real caring for her patients and they can perceive that. A lot of it is being able to talk about money without stumbling around."*

Tell Me Now

As you know, some patients want all the answers immediately, and they're not happy with postponing a conversation about treatment recommendations and fees. Your offer to study their case and know it by heart falls on deaf ears. When they press hard for answers, that is, if they ask more than once about specific treatment recommendations and fees, make your answer as direct as possible. This situation is common with out-of-town patients. Here's a typical conversation when the patient presses you for specifics. The patient is asking you to sell him the case. If you postpone your answer, you'll irritate your patient and create suspicion. Faced with this situation, here's a formula to follow:

- Give an overview of treatment.
- Give the prognosis of care.
- State the estimated fee.
- Estimate the total time in treatment and number of appointments.
- Ask whether this fits their budget and schedule.

Here's a sample dialogue. Your patient says: *"I know you have to plan my case, doc, but you've said you've done lots of cases like mine before. Give me an idea of what you'll do, how long it will take, and how much it will cost."*

You say: *"Mr. Humbert, I'm going to recommend that we rebuild all your back lower teeth, use implants with the upper teeth, and do cosmetic enhancements to your upper front teeth. As I said before, you've got good bone support and your gums are healthy, so we should get a great result. A case like yours will cost about 15,000 dollars and will take us about ten appointments over one year's time. Does that fit within your budget and schedule?"*

There are several typical responses to this hard-ball approach. Your patient might say yes. If so, then order your new boat! If the patient says, *"I had no idea it would be this expensive!"* a good response is:

"That's why I asked if it would fit into your budget. Your care doesn't need to be done all at once. Let me study your care and in the meantime, think about your annual budget, and I guarantee you, your care can be done within your budget over time."

When you bring the topic of budget up before the patient does, it gives you the right to refer to your previous comments about budget if the patient objects to the fees. It's much more powerful and insightful to anticipate the fee objection than to react to it.

For example, the patient might say, "Oh, my God, I had no idea dentistry was so expensive," or "You've got to be kidding—15,000 dollars just for teeth!" Your response to these and just about all fee objections is, "I understand. That's why I suggested you think about your budget."

Don't Hide from the Fee

Conversations about money need to be handled *exquisitely well*. Remember one major rule: *Don't make patients wrong about their attitude about money*. For example, many of us learned not to use certain words related to fees, words such as expensive, expense, costs, or money. We learned to say things like: "The *investment* in your dental health will be 5,000 dollars" or "This dentistry isn't expensive, it's an *investment* in your dental health" or "The *professional fee* for your care is 5,000 dollars."

When a patient says, "Wow, that's expensive," why say things like, "Compared to what?" and consequently, start a contest about what's expensive and what isn't? Why make patients wrong if they think dentistry is expensive? Converting a word like "expense" to "investment" is the oldest sales trick in the world and everyone knows it. Don't use euphemisms with patients. Talk in simple, straight, laymen's language—money, expense, costs. When I hear a salesman convert the word "cost" to "investment" I put my hand on my wallet. Don't hide from the fee.

Acknowledge that many patients believe that dentistry is expensive, and then move on and encourage patients to work within their budgets.

Rich Patients

I've had clients ask: "Won't my wealthy patients be insulted if I suggest my work may be outside their budget?" If you want to make your wealthy patients mad, assume that money is no object for them. Many of them are wealthy because they know how to manage and talk about money. Show them you do, too, and they'll respect you for it.

Just Say Yes

Since I wrote *Dentists: An Endangered Species* and have given many seminars on the topic of case acceptance of complete dentistry, I've had some dentists say, "I don't get into this budget thing like you do. If people want it, they'll find the money. I just quote the fee and most patients say yes."

Perhaps you've seen this happen in your practice, and I've heard several celebrity dentists make similar remarks. The fact is that most of us are not celebrity dentists, and sticker shock is one thing that most practices cannot afford. After you've logged a few hundred complete cases under your belt, you'll have the charisma, charm, and confidence to sell snowballs to Eskimos.

The trick is selling the first few hundred cases. The budget approach (CD-3) I've outlined in this chapter is the most direct, nonmanipulative, easy-to-learn technique to avoid the sticker shock that can embarrass and anger patients. In addition, your anxiety will ease when quoting high fees. You'll find, like the hundreds of dentists who are using this budget/schedule-based approach, that when you're more comfortable with high fees, you patients will be, too.

Reinforcing CD-3

After you've finished your conversation, reappoint the patient. Train your staff, including your receptionist, to reinforce CD-3: *"Mr. Humbert, next time Dr. Homoly will talk to you about your care. Be thinking about what's good for your budget and schedule. He's really good about staying within both."*

Personality Profiles

Many dentists ask me if I vary my approach based on patients' personalities. I'm also asked if I spend much time understanding the patients' concerns, hot buttons, and motivators, and then feed those concerns and motivators back to patients in order to influence them. Using personality profiles and hot buttons can work in the traditional case acceptance process, especially when you're communicating dental care to a nontarget patient, one who is not compelled to have his teeth fixed.

However, when dealing with the complete rehabilitative case, you can use personality profiles and hot button techniques, but if they're not ready, these techniques can disconnect you, and in particular, become visible as selling techniques and trigger anger in your patients. If target patients can't afford the care, or are surprised, embarrassed, or angered by your fee, no personality style or hot button will overcome their sticker shock. I'm not against personality profiling or delving into their concerns and motivators. In the big picture of selling complete care, these are small issues compared to their readiness and the fee.

If you can recognize readiness and handle the issues of fees, budgets, and schedules in the complete cases, then personality issues and motivators seem to work out through good listening skillls, intuition, and common sense.

The Spectrum of Appeal

Let's use the *Spectrum of Appeal* to look at fees. (See figure 1.) The fee, the dollar amount of the case, is a number and numbers are blue spectrum. However, a budget is a personal relationship with money, which moves into the red spectrum. If you think of fees only in terms of a dollar amount, you're missing an essential opportunity to create appeal. By showing you're aware and sensitive to budgets, you create red spectrum appeal to the patient.

Dr. Jay Crawford of Lansing, Michigan, says, *"Addressing the issue of the patient's budget early in the new patient process frees up the conversation about money. Money can be a battle ground. No longer. The single most important pearl I've used in case presentation is getting the budget issues out in the open early."*

If you ignore budgets and relate to patients with a lack of understanding and sensitivity to their budgets, at best you'll turn them off, and probably make them angry with you.

FIGURE 1: Fees vs. budget.

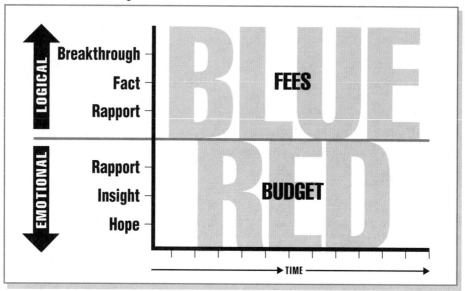

At lower levels, fees can be blue spectrum. However as the fees pass a certain point they become an emotional issue. (See figure 2.) Where this occurs depends on your patient. CD-3 begins the process of discovering where the crossover point from blue to red is. Most patients don't know or haven't thought about the crossover point and CD-3 plants the seed for that conversation at the next appointment.

There's a crossover point, from blue to red that affects the dentist and team members. It's the point that the fee becomes so large that you're hesitant to quote it. Your blue spectrum objectivity crosses over into red spectrum fear, which includes fear of creating an angry patient, fear of not knowing what to say when the patient screams "No way," and fear of rejection. CD-3 begins the process of easing the fear of quoting fees by making you aware of the patient's budget and comfort zone. When you know what patients are comfortable with financially, you'll feel much more comfortable recommending treatment that you know they can afford.

FIGURE 9: The fee crossover point.

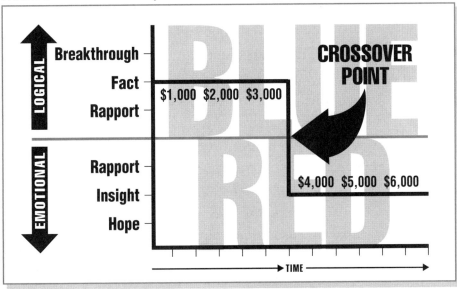

Dr. Gary Radz of Denver, Colorado, says: *"Back when you and I first started working together I was an associate in a practice that was charging $1,000 per crown. If I were the patient it would take me a year to pay for a crown. I wasn't making more than $40,000/$50,000 a year, had big student loans, and was presenting treatment to patients for 15,000 to 18,000 thousand dollars. I always had a big mental block of presenting any treatment than I couldn't pay for myself. I placed my financial situation and my value situation in my patients. Learning to recognize that I was doing that was a breakthrough.*

Just because I can't afford it doesn't mean they can't afford it. Once I figured that out, talking about big cases became easier and more patients went along with my recommendations."

StorySelling and CD-3

Critical Dialogue Number Three foreshadows the budget: "I'm really good about staying within a budget if I know I need to. Have you thought about your budget at all?"

StorySelling CD-3 talks about other patients who were concerned about finances or time, and how you identified their budget, including time, and completed their dentistry within their budget and schedule.

For example, you're asked: *"My budget? No, I haven't thought of any budget. Is this expensive?"* You say:

"Most of my patients are concerned about cost. In fact, cost was a major concern for Joe, a carpenter we have in the practice. Early in our relationship, Joe let me know what he was comfortable with, and we only did the dentistry that was within his budget. We'll do the same for you."

Become really good at telling stories about other patients who had concerns about costs because when you offer high-fee complete care dentistry, you'll often hear that concern.

You may believe it's impossible to ask honest questions and receive honest answers about a patient's budget. Most of us believe that when we start to talk about actual dollar amounts, any amount will be too much. Fortunately, we can determine a patient's dental budget and plan a schedule without embarrassing ourselves or the patient. In the next chapter you'll learn how to take yes for an answer.

CHAPTER 15

MISSION
Impossible

Discovering the Patient's Dental Budget

Isn't it frustrating when you present a terrific treatment plan, just to watch it unravel because you don't have the one critical piece of information that most often decides the fate of your plan—the patient's budget? Wouldn't it be great if you knew, *before* recommending care, what your patient's budget is? It's not "Mission Impossible" to discover what our patients' financial comfort zone is.

The information in this chapter takes you through the process of learning what's appropriate for your patient's budget and schedule relative to their lifetime strategy for dental health. Its goal is to take the sticker shock, embarrassment, and anger out of the case acceptance process, and recommend only that dentistry that falls within your patient's budget. Plus, this process does wonders for your mental health.

After the diagnostic appointment and the diagnostic material are assembled, reappoint the patient and present the treatment plan for the patient's lifetime strategy for dental health. Devise a treatment plan to the highest level of your clinical capacity, which with complete care cases, often includes teamwork with specialists. Don't break the plan into "good," "better," or "best" plans. The multiple plan approach works well in dental school where the goal is to demonstrate an understanding of multiple approaches to care, but it can be confusing and self-defeating in private practice.

Resist putting together multiple treatment plans using different combinations of restorations and fees.

Once complete, think through the treatment plan as if you were to do it in stages: quadrants, sextants, or arches. I found that the best way to do the case over time was by dividing partially edentulous cases into sextants: mandibular anterior, maxillary anterior, mandibular posterior, maxillary posterior. Fully edentulous cases can, at times, be divided into arches, maxillary and mandibular.

Now assign your treatment fee to each segment. The goal here is to anticipate the patient's budget limitations. Because most patients have budget restraints, you want to be able to offer the best care and associated fees spread out over time.

After the treatment plan and fees are determined, the patient returns for the case preview and case discussion during the same appointment.

Case Preview

In *Dentists: An Endangered Species* I labeled the "Case Preview" the "Case Review." After teaching this principle for many years, I've come to realize that this principle is best understood as a preview, not a review.

The case preview gives the patient an idea of what treatment is possible within the guidelines of his schedule and budget. It's like a preview of coming attractions at the theater. If he likes what he sees and hears, he can proceed. Critical Dialogue Number Four (CD-4) occurs within the case preview.

Critical Dialogue Number Four

The case preview occurs about a week or so after the patient's diagnostic appointment. Your patient is seated in the treatment area. Tell her you'd like to take a look at a few things before you talk. Your dental assistant should anticipate Golden Moments as she seats the patient.

The structure of the case preview is to present the lifetime strategy for dental health to the patient in the *future tense* by saying, "Here's what could be done if it's right for your schedule and budget." This conversation is CD-4. It's like saying, "We can go to Disneyland if you want to and have the time and money."

After the patient is in the chair, lean her back, take a look, and, while examining her mouth, start you presentation. You want the case discussion to be an unstructured moment. Speak as if you're thinking out loud. Occasionally, roll your stool back and talk directly to the patient. Your attitude and tone of voice conveys a "thinking out loud" tone, not the tone used while making a formal presentation. The case preview is not a dialogue between you and your patient; it's a monologue. You don't want to get into a question-and-answer session now. The case preview is a preview of coming attractions, reminding your patient that you're not making firm recommendations, but giving her an idea of what's possible if it works for her budget and schedule.

Here's a typical case preview CD-4 monologue:

"Mrs. Slingerland, before we talk about your care there are a few things I'd like to look at again.

"I know you're disappointed with the discomfort and movement of your lower partial denture. We could use dental implants to give you permanent teeth that you'd brush right in your own mouth. Of course, when we do that depends on your budget and schedule. I know you're a busy person.

"The missing upper back teeth could be replaced with perma-nent teeth, just like you had when you were sixteen.

"You've told me several times that you don't like the way your front teeth look. When you're ready, we can put a thin, porcelain tooth-colored coating on them, just like you saw in the pictures in the brochures."

Now, sit the patient up, and tell your assistant to bring Mrs. Slingerland to the talking area: *"I know you have some questions. Suzette will take you up front where we can talk."*

Notice how the language of CD-4 focuses on future possibilities, using verbs like "could," "can," "will," and the phrase, "when you're ready." Become good at saying, "when you're ready." It lets the patient know what's possible but gives her control. In CD-4 *never* say, "Here's the best treatment for you," or "This is state-of-the-art dentistry," or "We're definitely going to Disneyland."

Now get out of the operatory ASAP and create a wonderful opportunity for a Golden Moment between your assistant and the patient. In fact, this is probably the *most* important Golden Moment. The patient has heard the coming attractions and chances are excellent she'll ask your assistant one or all of the following questions: *"How much does all this cost?" "Will this hurt?" "How will I look when we're all done?" "How many cases like mine do you do?" "Do I really need all this work?"* This is an exquisite unstructured selling opportunity. Anticipate and excel in it.

Seat the patient in your consultation area (I call it the "talking area" to maintain its informality). Don't rush to join the patient. Let Golden Moments happen. Your assistants will tell you when it's time for you. The case preview (CD-4) is complete after you've given the patient the preview of coming attractions. Our next step is the case discussion.

Case Discussion and Critical Dialogue Number Five

Case discussion is the explanation of the dental care that falls within the patient's budget and schedule. We want to recommend only that care that that fits within his budget. In order to do this, you have to know what the budget is! The good news is that you're closer to knowing the patient's budget than you think.

Absolutely do not get into a step-by-step explanation of what you're going to do and why. Do not show before and after wax-ups, or go into a show-and-tell technical discussion. Case discussion is not informed consent. Read chapter 10 to refresh your memory. Let the patient talk and answer only those questions you're asked. You'll provide consent at another time, but not now.

After the assistant tells you your patient is ready, enter your talking area and immediately ask: *"Did our discussion a few minutes ago make sense? Was I clear as I was giving you some ideas about our care?"* Get the patient talking and don't start with technical explanations.

The patient naturally begins to ask treatment questions: *"What is an implant?" "What do you mean when you say you'll put porcelain coatings on my front teeth?" "How many caps do I need?"* Give short answers to these treatment questions using visual language as much as possible. After the patient asks a few treatment questions, shift the focus of your conversation from clinical to budget issues.

Patients may ask an administrative question, such as "How long will this take?" and "How much will it cost?" or "How much will my insurance pay?" If this happens, direct your conversation to the budget issues.

> **The goal of case discussion is to determine the budget, and if you get too deep into clinical issues this conversation will lose focus.**

An important reminder: You absolutely must stay connected during conversations about money. (Study chapter 3.) If you're not confident about your communication skills, the case discussion will be uncomfortable for both you and the patient.

After you've answered a few clinical questions or when the patient asks an administrative question, remind him of the promise made in CD-3. *"I'm really good about staying within your budget if I know I need to. Have you thought at all about your budget?"* You've guaranteed your patient that you'd provide only that dentistry that will fit the patient's budget. Now it's time to revisit your promise.

Here's an example of CD-5. The patient has just finished asking her second clinical question or asks an administrative question.

"Mrs. Campbell, these are great questions, but before I make any firm recommendations for care, I need to know how much of this will fit within your budget and schedule. Remember last time I asked you to think about your budget? Give me an idea of what you're comfortable with and let's do only the dentistry that will fit within it."

Now, remain silent and let the patient talk. Keep CD-5 short. Don't explain why you're asking it—the reason is obvious. Any talking you do now results from your discomfort, not the patient's. Remember, treatment suitability is based largely on the patient's budget and schedule.

Patient Responses

When you deliver CD-5, the most common responses are:

- "I don't know what my budget is."
- "Tell me what I need and I'll tell you if it fits my budget."
- "I don't have a budget for dentistry."

Expect over 95 percent of patients to give you one of these responses, so get good at dealing with them. When you hear any of these responses, follow them with a direct statement that gives them:

- The total fee for the lifetime strategy of dental health.
- The total time it will take to complete it.
- The question, "Does that fit within your budget?"

For example, you say to your patient:

"Wanda, give me an idea of what you're comfortable with and let's do only the dentistry that will fit within it."

"I don't know about budgets for dental care," Wanda replies. *"I've always gone to the dentist and he's told me what I needed and the receptionist told me how much it costs. How much does all this work cost?"*

"Wanda, your total treatment fee is 5,000 dollars and will take us about six months to compete. Are you comfortable with that?"

Notice that we're right back where we started, "What is your budget?" This encourages the patient to rethink her budget in light of the new information she has—the total fee and time for a lifetime strategy.

Expect one of two responses from Wanda—yes or no.

Let's start with no. When you hear it, assume it's in response to the fee, not to the dentistry. Do not assume patients don't want the dentistry just because it's not in their budget. Your job is to help them find a way to fit the care into their budget. Most dentists, when they hear a fee objection, change the treatment. Don't. They're not objecting to the dentistry, they're objecting to the fee. Become good at making that distinction.

After you hear no, follow with suggestions about ways to spread the treatment over time. Recommend specific dollar amounts over a period of time and give them an idea of how long it will take to complete their care by working within a budget. Then revisit the issue of budget again.

For example, you say:

"Wanda, your total treatment fee is 5,000 dollars and will take us about six months to compete. Will that fit within your budget?"

"No, doctor, I had no idea it would be that expensive."

"Wanda, that's why I suggested you stay within your budget. A good way to do your care is over time. If you're comfortable with a budget of 2500 dollars a year, we'll have you finished in two years. Does that work better for you"?

Notice I immediately reminded Wanda that I suggested she think about (stay within) her budget. Almost always the best response to fee objections is, *"That's why I suggested you stay within your budget."* This response reminds the patient that you want to work within their budget. It also keeps you from having to defend your fees, treatment plan, and your ethics. If you have not suggested that she think about her budget (CD-3), then it's less credible to suggest budgeting her care.

Dr. John Howard of Savannah, Georgia has a wonderful attitude when discussing fees. When patients express concerns about his fees, he assures them by saying: *"This is important dentistry for you and we've got to find a way to help you get your teeth fixed."*

I love the "we've got to find a way" part of his response. It puts him and the patient on the same side of the chair. John is overwhelmingly successful in making his patients comfortable during case presentation because he knows how to talk about money without embarrassing or angering patients.

If your budget recommendations remain unacceptable to the patient, and you're unable to suggest a budget to be implemented over time, then return to the chief complaint in CD-2. Recommend that you fix the chief complaint only, and when the patient is ready, proceed with a lifetime strategy.

For example, you say:

"Wanda, a good way to do your care is over time. If you're comfortable with a budget of 2500 dollars a year, we can have you finished in two years. Does that work better for you?"

"Oh, no. I couldn't make that work at all. What else can you do?"

"Wanda, would a budget of a 1,000 dollars make it possible for you to start your care?"

"No, it just seems like it's too much to spend."

"Wanda, I understand. Let me make this recommendation. Let's fix that black front tooth you're worried about and stay within your budget, and when you're ready to fix the rest of your teeth, I'll be glad to help you."

Returning to the chief complaint is an excellent way for you to keep the door open. Patients' budgets and circumstances change. Don't make them wrong or pressure them. Don't make a contest out of case acceptance. If your patients aren't ready, give them a way to feel good about staying in your practice, and when they're ready, they'll say so.

Take "Yes" for an Answer

When you hear "yes" to: *"Wanda, your total treatment fee is 5,000 dollars and will take us about six months to compete. Will that fit within your budget?"*(or subsequent budget recommendations), begin the financial arrangement process. Call your financial coordinator into the talking area and explain to her, in front of your patient, what the issues are and how they will be handled.

For example, your patient says:

"Yes, doctor, 2,500 dollars a year will work out okay."

"Wanda, let me get Ginger in here and she can help us get started."

Ginger enters. *"Ginger, Wanda has decided to go ahead with her lifetime strategy for dental health. Her total treatment fee is 5,000 dollars and we're going to be doing it over two years, 2,500 dollars per year. Wanda, our normal financial arrangements for your first year's work are one-third of the fee due next time, another third is due at the middle of treatment, and the last third is due when we're done.*

"Ginger, it will take us about two months to complete Wanda's care. Give her the information about consent for treatment, and her next appointment will be twenty minutes.

"Wanda, Ginger is going to give you information about the risks, benefits, and alternatives to care that dental ethics and state law requires me to provide. Next time we'll review this material, I'll answer any questions you have, and we'll start

your care. Read this information and if you have any questions, just underline them or call me.

To Ginger: *"Wanda understands that she'll pay us directly and her insurance company will reimburse her.*

"Wanda, did you have any questions for me while Ginger is here?" (Respond to questions).

It's important that you have this dialogue in front of your patient and your financial coordinator so if any loose ends unravel, you're there to deal with them. Don't leave the room until everyone is on the same page.

The financial coordinator at Dr. John and Julie Howard's office, Lawannda, says: *"It's comforting to know that when they've finished with a case presentation, not only has the patient accepted treatment, but the patient is also now financially committed in the way we have designed. Our accounts receivable are under control now and we're moving away from financing our patients in-house. That's allowed us to really feel confident that in the next six to twelve months that our dream of having no in-house billing at all will come true! We're able to treat the new patients according to their chief complaints and budgets, which makes it easy to create a more predictable financial arrangement with them."*

Make your financial coordinator's job easy by clearly and confidently stating the particulars about the plan, finances, and your understanding with the patient.

Yes, I Do Have a Budget

Occasionally, after you've asked your patient to think about his budget (CD-3), and you ask what it is (CD-5), the patient states a budgeted dollar amount. This is rare, but it does happen. This budget is either above or below your fee for the lifetime strategy for dental health. Let's start with a budget below your fee.

If the budget is below your fee, assume the budget is an annual amount and divide the total fee into the annual budget, and recommend that the patient extend treatment time and stay within his budget. Stay positive and look for ways to support the patient in his budget decision.

For example, your patient's fee is 12,000 dollars. In response to CD-5 he says:

"Yeah, doc, I thought about it. I can't spend more than 4000 dollars. Can you do it for that?"

"We can get a good start on it for that. In year one I'll fix your upper and lower front teeth. In year two, we'll replace your missing lower back teeth. And in year three, we'll replace your missing upper back teeth. We'll have you finished in three years and stay within your budget."

Notice that I did not start a contest about the budget. Instead I went with what the patient said and made the case work over time. I made the patient right, not wrong, about his budget.

The Best Question in Dentistry

When you divide the budget into the total fee and spread the treatment out over time, some interesting dialogues occur. Many of these dialogues circle right back to the original question of budget. It's important to notice that I am not playing games with the patient. I'm taking her budget seriously and encouraging her to stay within it.

For example, your patient's fee is 15,000 dollars. In response to CD-5 she says:

"Yes, my budget is 3,000 dollars. Can you do it for that?"

"We can get a good start on it for that. In year one I'll fix your lower front teeth. In year two, we'll fix your upper front teeth. In year three, fix your lower back teeth. Year four, fix your upper back teeth on the right. And year five, fix the other side. We'll have you finished in five years and stay within your budget."

"You mean it's going to take me five years to get my teeth fixed?"

"Yes," you say, "and we'll stay within your budget. Is that what you'd like to do?"

"Well, how long would it take if we did the whole thing?"

"Your total care is 15,000 dollars and if we did it all at once, I could have you finished within three months. Does that work for you?"

The patient's question, *"Well, how long would it take if we did the whole thing?"* is the best question in dentistry because it's the best indicator that the patient is ready for care and is looking for a way to do it. Your answer should state the total fee and the total time in treatment. Then return to the issue of budget— "Does that work for you?" If the patient indicates the total fee is outside his annual budget, then return to the offer of treatment over time.

For example, you say:

"Your total care is 15,000 dollars and if we did it all at once, I could have you finished within three months. Does that work for you?"

"There's no way I can afford 15,000 dollars. What else can you do?"

"Let's stay within your budget. Let's do your care over time. If you're comfortable with a 3,000 dollar budget, then let's start there."

The choice you're asking the patient to make is total care versus total care over time, instead of total care versus no care. Using this approach, you'll find yourself doing a lot of big cases spread over time. Would you rather do two cases for 5,000 dollars or no cases for 10,000 dollars?

Yeah, But … Versus Yes, And …

Often when you're breaking the case down into years, the patient interrupts and objects to the time over which treatment would be spread. The temptation is to blame the budget and justify your position. Don't. Instead, affirm their budget decision and be cheerful about it.

When you blame the budget for extended treatment times it sounds like, *"Yeah, but your budget is only 3000 dollars and if we're going to do your case for that budget it means five years in treatment."* When you affirm the budget and remain cheerful it sounds like: *"Yes, and you'll be able to get exactly the dentistry you want and stay within your budget."*

Let the patient argue with his budget. Agree to that budget and do the case over time. If the budget isn't feasible, then return to the chief complaint.

This technique works well when the patient says: *"My budget is what my insurance will pay."* Keep in mind that the "insurance only" patient usually never gets this far into the process. He usually opts for the chief complaint in CD-2. If one slips through to CD-5, then use the treatment over time approach. After realizing that insurance will never pay for his care, return to the budget issue, without blaming insurance or making the patient wrong for wanting to use it.

For example, your patient's total fee is 11,000 dollars and he says:

"My budget is what my insurance will pay. Can you do it for that?"

"I'll try. In year one I'll fix this one tooth. Year two, we'll fix the one next to it. In year three…"

"Wait a minute, doc. At that rate it's going to take me a decade to fix my teeth."

"Yes, and we'll stay within your budget. Is that what you'd like to do?"

"I guess my insurance stinks. How much would it be if we did the whole thing?"

"Your total fee is 11,000 dollars and will take us about six months to complete. Does that fit within your budget?"

From here, follow the pathways to an annual budget over time, and have the insurance company reimburse the patient.

Dr. Gary Radz says: *"I had a patient who needed a great amount of work, and her previous dentist had not addressed the aesthetics she was concerned about. After we spoke and I examined her, I said, 'I have an idea about what you want, and I can do all the work for you—probably better than you imagine is possible. So when you come back for you next visit I'll need an idea about your budget. I want to stay within the amount you want to want to spend and still give you the results you're looking for.'*

My patient looked me straight in the eye and said, 'I have 10,000 dollars I've been saving—took me more than two years. That's what I've got to spend.'

Even though, her total cost would probably be about 14,000 dollars, I knew were in the ballpark, and I knew she was interested enough to spend the money. When she came back I assured her that I could do the work and stay within the initial budget, but I also added that by spending just a little more, she could get an even better result. I couldn't have had that conversation if I hadn't been up front about the money. We can lay out all kinds of options to patients—like a car salesman who starts throwing in the options and they're adding up totals in their heads—but all the patient is thinking about is how much it's going to cost. Once you get the money issue out in the open, you can find out if you're in the same ballpark."

Fake Budgets

During my seminars I always hear at least one participant say: "Patients aren't going to tell you what they can afford. They'll lowball you, seeing if you'd cave in. How do you know they're giving you their real budget?"

It doesn't matter if it's their real budget. If it isn't, and after you've done a great job doing their initial dentistry, they'll suggest that you do the rest of the work, forget the first budget, and you're a happy dentist. If it is, and you respect it, and do a great job on their initial work, they'll refer like crazy to you and you're a hero!

Assume the budget they give you is real and respect it.

[243]

"I've Got the Money"

When the patient tells you his budget is greater than or equal to your total fee, proceed directly to financial arrangements. This occurs most often when the patient is a spouse of a high-fee patient and aware of the fees. "Doc, my wife's case cost 10,000 dollars. I figure mine would be about the same." Lucky you!

Patient Financing

I'm often asked if I think patient financing is a good idea. I like the idea of helping patients afford dentistry. Budget issues are easier to deal with if there is an outside third party involved. I never recommend that the dentist carry the debt, with the patients making payments to the office. There are excellent patient financing companies that can support your patients.

One caution related to patient financing is that debt can turn a clinical problem into a management problem. Chances are excellent you'll have a clinical issue with advanced rehabilitative cases: porcelain fracture, endodontic flare-ups, recurring periodontal issues, material failure or fracture. These events are disappointing to patients and when they are still paying on work that your now repairing, for a fee, a simple endodontic procedure can escalate into a contest. Working with outside financing helps to prevent contests.

Get Out of the Corner

Financial conversations often make my clients feel as if they're being backed into a corner. Two things push dentists into corners: answering questions/objections about fees and what to say when the patient says no.

> **The best response to fee objections, no matter how strong, is the offer to stay within the patient's budget.**

Fee objections may occur at any point in the relationship with the patient and are not limited to CD-5 dialogues. Patients may voice fee objections on the telephone, during the examination, while having radiographs taken, or in the hallway on the way to the front desk. The best responses to fee objections deflect the objection to the position of budget.

Examples of fee objections:

1. Receptionist on telephone—*"I understand your concern about costs. Dr. Jarvis is excellent about staying within your budget."*
2. Chair-side assistant taking radiographs—*"I guarantee you Dr. Allen will work within your budget and schedule."*
3. Hygienist at initial appointment—*"You'll appreciate how Dr. Misch works within your budget."*
4. Scheduler at front desk—*"Dr. Severance will work with your budget. He's great at that."*

Don't sound like a broken record when offering to work within your patient's budget. Remember, budget is money *and* time. Vary your delivery—refer to money and time alternatively. Stay out of the corner on fee objections; offer to work within the budget.

"One of the best things I learned is to just be up front about money...
I need to know what kind of budget they've got planned for this kind of work... It's like looking for a house. I can find you any kind of house you want, but I need to know what you can afford to spend."
Lori Tuttle, Office Administrator

Taking "No" for an Answer

Not knowing what to say when the patients say no is the second thing that pushes dentists into corners. This leaves an awkward silence and creates stress for everyone. When it becomes obvious that a patient is not ready or doesn't have the budget, say: *"Maybe, Mr. Crawford, this is not a good time to get your teeth fixed. When you're ready we'll be here."* This response leaves the door open and doesn't make the patient wrong or embarrassed.

Accepting no for an answer is tough to do. We've been trained to go for yes. Many seminars teach that no is not an option. Keep in mind we're not selling soap, cars, insurance, or stereos. I'm all for learning sales techniques from sales professionals, but it cuts both ways. They need to learn from us that pushing people to say yes makes you sound like a salesman. And salesmen don't sell complete dentistry. Taking no for an answer is part of selling complete dentistry.

StorySelling and CD-4 and CD-5

Critical dialogue numbers four and five occur during the case preview and case discussion. Be ready to StorySell a wide variety of issues. I've already listed the toughest questions you'll answer. Because CD-5 is the dialogue in which the patient commits to treatment, be prepared to tell YourStory and stories about how other patients overcame similar objections. You'll discover that once you've developed five or six great stories, you can use them interchangeably, depending on the topic. You don't need a separate story for each objection or comment.

The Wedding Dress

Imagine you're a twenty-five year-old woman and you and your bridesmaids are shopping for a wedding dress. You walk into a bridal showroom and the saleswoman whisks you up, takes you to the fitting area, and hands you a snow white gown in a clear vinyl bag. You slip it on, you pose on the fitting platform; you look into the mirror and see that it's perfect. It's better than perfect. It's everything any woman has ever dreamed of and more. Your bridesmaids clutch their hands and sigh. Then you notice a little yellow tag hanging from the elbow. You read it and it says 15,000 dollars. For an instant you hope that it's a terrible mistake, but in a heartbeat more, you realize that this dress can never be yours. Your bridesmaids freeze, and while they watch your eyes become liquid, the dark cloud of your budget casts its long shadow.

"I had no idea this dress was so expensive," you gasp to the sales lady.

"Well if it's more than you can spend, let's go over to the bargain rack and see what's left."

Your wedding will never be the same. You were so close but so far away.

When we don't have an idea of our patient's budgets, we put many of them in the position of being so close, but so far away.

Take time to discover what is appropriate for you patients' budgets. Don't let the long dark shadow of their budget dim your relationship. If patients have budget issues, discover them early, and make it acceptable to work within the budget. You'll do a lot more complete care dentistry when you can handle budget issues smoothly.

FIGURE 1: Case preview/case discussion.

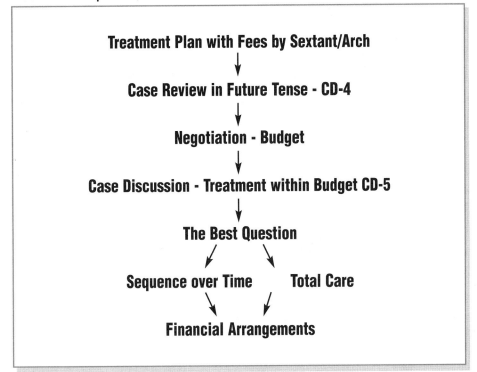

CHAPTER 16

On Your Mark,
GET SET,
Don't Go

The Preoperative Appointment

You've just sold a big case. Now, a week later, it's Monday morning and you've got three hours scheduled to start your big case. The first half of her fee is due, 4,000 dollars, and you're ready to go. At 8:15 the patient calls and cancels because "she's sick." Now you're sick. Your staff runs and hides from you and you feel like you're all dressed up with nowhere to go. Know the feeling?

Nothing is worse than a false start because you lose time and money. "On your mark, get set, don't go" is no way to live. If you want to preserve your mental health and collection goals, learn to structure the preoperative appointment.

The preoperative appointment is part of the case acceptance process. It's the short, usually twenty minute, appointment following the case preview/case discussion. Its goal is to confirm that the patient is really going to start treatment. Just because patients have agreed to everything does not mean that they'll follow through. But you already know that, so why it is that we're surprised or disappointed when patients "don't go." Usually it's because we find out it's "don't go" when they cancel their initial long appointment. Why do they cancel? Usually money is the issue; they don't have the first part of their fee. So when they cancel you lose the money *and* the time. You can make up the money, but you can't get the time back. The solution? Don't attach a big fee to a long appointment.

The preoperative appointment is designed to provide informed consent, collect the first portion of the fee, and to begin care.

Set the Stage

A big part of the success of the preoperative appointment results from the stage set in the previous appointment, the case preview/case discussion. Do you remember the conversation I had with my patient Wanda in front of my financial coordinator Ginger? Here it is for review.

"Ginger, Wanda has decided to go ahead with her lifetime strategy for dental health. Her total treatment fee is 5,000 dollars and we're going to be doing it over two years, 2,500 dollars

per year. Wanda, our normal financial arrangements for your first year's work is that one-third of the fee is due next time, another third is due at the middle of treatment, and the last third is due when we're done. Ginger, it will take us about two months to complete Wanda's care."

"Give her the information about consent for treatment, and her next appointment will be twenty minutes. Wanda, Ginger is going to give you information about the risks, benefits, and alternatives to care that state law requires me and by dental ethics to do. Next time we'll review this material, I'll answer any questions you have, and we'll start your care. Read this information and if you have any questions, just underline them or call me. Wanda understands that she'll pay us directly and her insurance company will reimburse her. Wanda, did you have any questions for me while Ginger is here? (Respond to questions.) *Ginger, do you have any questions for me?"* (Respond to questions.)

I leave the room following this dialogue with Wanda, at which point Ginger confirms that Wanda understands, gives her consent forms, answers questions, and sets the next appointment. It's between the case preview/case discussion appointment and the preoperative appointment that the patient is sent the case discussion letter. This is a very important step.

The Case Discussion Letter

When was the last time you received a letter from your physician outlining what you needed to do to maintain a life strategy of medical health? When was the last time any of your patients received a letter from their previous dentist outlining the requirements of maintaining a lifetime of dental health? I'll bet you never received such a letter.

If you want to sell complete dentistry you have to differentiate yourself from the rest of the pack.

Your patient receives the case discussion letter within three to four days following your case preview/discussion. It's the one thing that most dentists won't do, and yet it is one of the best ways to differentiate yourself.

In chapter 7 of *Dentists: An Endangered Species*, I went into great detail about the structure and function of this letter. Read it again if you have the book. Here's a quick summary. The case discussion letter:

- Adds value to your relationship with the patient.
- Organizes the sequence of care.
- Is a timely reminder of your treatment recommendations.
- Is accurate and neat, which signals the quality of your dentistry.
- Has a compounding affect over time.

Since I first wrote about it in 1996 in *Dentists: An Endangered Species,* clients who have started using the case discussion letter are experiencing its dramatic benefits. The short-term benefits are obvious. The letter is a valuable, unexpected positive experience that will set you apart from most dentists. See my web site at www.paulhomoly.com to order *Dentists: An Endangered Species*.

The long-term benefits are more valuable than the short-term benefits. Here's why. Most patients who receive this letter will start their treatment, but some will not. Although they may not start treatment, it's been my experience that they will save the letter. Over time you may have 100 or more patients who have delayed treatment but still have your letter and when they're ready, they'll be back. With 100 patients who have been through the case acceptance process and have accepted the lifetime strategy but have postponed treatment, chances are excellent you'll see one of these patients return to your practice each month. They'll have letter in hand and tell you, "I'm ready!" What would one new complete case a month mean to your practice? Probably 100,000 dollars a year.

> **Is 100,000 dollars a year worth the effort of writing an excellent case acceptance letter? You bet it is!**

Confirm the Fee

At least two days before the preoperative appointment confirm the appointment by phone, fax, and/or e-mail. Confirm the time, duration, and fee. When confirming appointments always confirm the fee.

Consent for Treatment

I've included examples of consent forms in *Dentists: An Endangered Species*. Re-read chapter 8 in *Dentists: An*

Endangered Species, in which I outline the flow and dialogues of the consent process.

I'm often asked if I offer alternatives to the lifetimes strategy: i.e., plan A, plan B, and plan C. I do not offer the good, better, best approach during case discussion, but I do during consent. Consent is where the alternatives belong. In fact consent is informed *only* when a patient is aware and understands alternatives to care. On occasion I will offer alternatives to care during case discussion. However, my strong preference is to offer time and budget options during case discussion and treatment options during consent.

What About Lawsuits?

When you practice complete dentistry, chances are excellent that eventually a patient will be unhappy with something you did, sue you, and try make the next two years of your life miserable. This is a fact of life; there's no escaping it. What we can do is take some preventive measures that will help stiff-arm legal challenges and boost mental health during the litigation process.

"Hello, Dr. Homoly. My name is Dr. Lucky and I was told by a friend to call you about a lawsuit that I'm in."

I hate getting these calls.

"What's going on?" I ask, hoping he'll hang up.

"Well, I had a patient who…" and the story weaves the details of the bad experiences and indignities. *"…and the reason I'm calling you is to see what you think about this whole mess."*

At times I can help callers with a referral to a great barracuda defense attorney, or by offering simple encouragement and practice management strategies to help the practice maintain an even keel during the storm of the lawsuit. Sometimes amateur marriage counseling is about all I can do!

Over the years I've been an expert witness for defendant dentists, heard dozens of lawsuit stories, and have had a few of my own. Here are some observations I have about the medial/ legal process.

Above all, a lawsuit is not about being right. So much of the suffering from a malpractice action is the indignity and the lack of basis for the accusation, which is that we are wrong. The suffering stems from the fact that we believe we are right and when we prove we are right, we will prevail. Wrong.

You can prove all day long you were right and still lose—ask me how I know.

The lawsuit is not about proving you're right. It's about money—your insurance company's money—and your perceived breach of standard of care is the path to this money. "Standard of care" is the legal window dressing added to the process of dental malpractice. Being right has nothing to do with it. Don't think for a heartbeat that a plaintiff's lawyer and his team of expert witnesses are in it to achieve justice.

The plaintiff's role is to distort "the facts" to support his claims, and the defense's role is to do the same. During this process, the real facts, being right, are lost while all the players jockey for position, and ultimately, the sympathy of a jury.

My advice to most dentists is to take an aggressive posture, return fire, and create as much stress as possible for the plaintiffs and their expert witnesses. The process does not support being right; the process supports and rewards whoever is the strongest and willing to go the distance.

Being right helps, but being strong helps more.

A major contributing factor to dental malpractice suits is the abundant availability of expert witnesses. Don't blame the lawyers alone for malpractice suits. By themselves they do not have the expert knowledge to defeat you. It's the hired expert witnesses for the plaintiff that are the real source of the leverage of the plaintiff's case. Did you know that there are dentists who actively market their testimony against other dentists to the legal profession? If you want to do something about the spread of dental malpractice challenges, do something about the "hired gun" expert witnesses.

Collect the Fee/ Start Care

Collect the fee after you've provided consent. Be very clear about when subsequent payments are due. After providing consent and collecting the fee, begin the care. Remember that this is a short appointment. Take a photograph, a shade, measure the facial dimensions, mouth opening, all of which get the ball rolling. The point here is to start the clinical process no matter how small the step. It serves as a strong emotional surge for patients because they know they are on their way to a lifetime strategy for dental health. It's a good feeling.

CHAPTER 17

With This Patient,
I Thee
Wed

The Team Approach to Case Acceptance

When two offices share the same patient, it's like getting married, hence, "With this patient, I thee wed." You're in it together, for better or worse. You're in the same boat, so you can't sink the half the others are in.

I help many dentists implement the team approach to complete care: two or more dentists in different offices, usually a specialist and a generalist, treating the same patient. Often a patient won't accept team treatment and that's when the battle starts between offices. At times I feel like a marriage counselor. Like the disgruntled partners in a marriage who are happy to confess all of their partner's sins but fail to see their role in their misery, members of the team often point the finger of blame while not understanding how they contribute to their own problems.

The team approach to dental care is not simple and is growing more complex as technology advances. However, the technical considerations are rarely the culprit when the team approach to care fails. Clearly the team approach fails most often because of conflicting messages the patient receives during the case acceptance process.

Just before starting a seminar I was approached by three periodontists. One of them cornered me.

"I'll tell you what's wrong with most general dentists I work with," he whined. "They're shot blockers. They 'un-sell' more dentistry than they sell. I'd starve if I had to rely on their referrals. They need to get their act together."

"Amen," cheered his buddies. "How do we get them to change?"

Later that day, a general dentist handed me a radiograph. It showed seven implants—two were failing and one was unrestorable. "I sent my patient to my oral surgeon for an implant evaluation. Nine months later the patient returned with a mouth full of implants and couldn't afford the restorative dentistry. What can I do to keep that from happening again?" he complained.

Disagreements, misunderstandings, and ambiguous situations concerning fees, insurance, methods of payment, scheduling, and bad attitudes lead the pack as reasons patients quit the treatment process before they get to first base. These conflicts are a result of weak relationships among team members, who call themselves a team, but they don't quite know how to act as a team. These relationships affect the entire team treatment process and the patient is caught in the middle.

> **Like children within a family, patients can either thrive or suffer depending on the relationship skills of those responsible for their care.**

The Honeymoon Is Over

Here is a typical team approach situation. A new patient comes into the general dentist's office. He examines the patient and concludes that the best way to replace the missing posterior teeth is to use dental implants. He explains this to the patient and recommends that she see an oral surgeon for implant evaluation.

If the general dentist is lucky, the patient will take his advice and seek the opinion of the specialist. Following the examination, the specialist describes the use of dental implants, shows the patient visual aids, and gives her a consent form to read at home. Just as the specialist is ready to escort the patient out the door, she asks the knockout question: *"How much will my insurance pay for this work?"*

The specialist winces. *"Didn't your general dentist explain all this to you?"*

"No," she says, *"the only thing he did was send me here and I'm not sure I can afford all this. How much does a reline cost?"*

Does this sound familiar? No wonder treatment teams talk about each other like battling married couples. Like children of conflicting parents, patients sense when teams are not in harmony.

Patients say yes to team treatment when they perceive the teams enjoy working with each other, communicate well, and have a good history.

Work and Harmony

It's important to make a distinction between teamwork and team harmony. Teamwork is the technical aspect to the team approach to care and includes copying records, duplicating radiographs, referral letters, follow-up telephone calls, and so forth. Teamwork is behind-the-scenes work, and patients may be unaware of the work the team is doing. Team harmony is characterized by the relationships that guide the team approach to care and is what the patient sees and experiences. Team harmony reveals itself in cheerful attitudes around team members, amiable communication, and collegiality.

To the patient, team harmony is more visible and has greater impact than teamwork.

The optimal team approach to case acceptance is a blend of teamwork and team harmony. The challenge within the team approach to case acceptance is to polish teamwork skills and constantly reinforce the value of the team—the team harmony. Let's revisit the scenario in which the new patient enters the general dentist's office. This time let's change the courtship sequence to case acceptance and apply the principles of case acceptance for complete care dentistry as outlined earlier.

The Six Steps

Chapter 7, which discussed structure, outlined the six steps in the structure of selling complete dentistry:

- Initial experience
- Diagnostic appointment
- Case preview
- Case discussion
- Case discussion letter
- Preoperative appointment

These six steps assume that the dentist is doing all aspects of care. In the team approach to care, in which general dentists are working with other general dentists or specialists, there are seven steps in the structure of selling high dollar dentistry. I've indicated in which office each step is completed:

- Initial experience — GP
- Diagnostic appointment — GP
- Case preview — GP
- Case discussion — GP
- Referral — Specialist
- Case discussion letter — GP and specialist
- Preoperative appointment — GP and specialist

The team approach to case acceptance includes the following steps for the general dentist. The general dentist:

- builds a solid relationship with the patient.
- determines if the patient is interested in minor dental care or comprehensive care involving specialty procedures (CD-2).
- explains the comprehensive treatment plan for the patient (including the time and fees for specialty procedures).
- determines the patient's annual budget for dental care (CD-3, CD-4).
- communicates the plan and recommends that portion of the plan that falls within the patient's budget (CD-5).

Building Solid Relationships

The team approach to case acceptance begins by determining if the patient is interested in treating his chief complaint only or in devising a lifetime strategy for dental health (CD-2). The traditional team approach to care occurs when a general dentist spots something that is out of his/her area of technical training, and refers the patient to a specialist. But the traditional approach is flawed! The role of the general dentist in the team approach is to act as the *anchor* office. If the referral is made too soon without building a relationship, the patient does not have support in place to enter into complex care. Patients rely on their general dentists to help them make decisions about the recommendations of the specialist. Instead of offering immediate referral, build the relationship with the patient. It's naive to think the patient can have two quality relationships (the team approach) before she has one (with the general dentist's office).

The foundation of the team approach to care is the patient having a solid relationship with the general dentist's office.

If the patient opts for a comprehensive lifetime approach to dental health, the general dentist's office performs a complete examination, collects all diagnostic tools (mounted study models, photographs, and so forth), and develops a complete treatment plan. In the team approach to care, the general dentist must have an overall understanding of the specialist's fees and treatment criteria. This knowledge allows the general dentist to estimate fees and treatment time for specialist procedures the general dentist doesn't perform but recommends to the patient. The estimates for fees and time in treatment for specialty procedures do not have to be exact. In fact, it's better to err on the liberal side of treatment fees and time in treatment when estimating specialty procedure treatment.

Determining the Patient's Annual Budget

During the examination and diagnostic appointments the general dentist and the patient are building a relationship that will become the basis for the referral. Part of this relationship is about learning the patient's annual budget for dental care (CD-3). The budget discussion is introduced (CD-3) and at the following appointment the budget is determined (CD-4).

Communicating the Treatment Plan

Once the budget is determined, the lifetime strategy treatment plan is offered in segments designed to stay within the patient's budget (CD-5). This budget may or may not be sufficient to complete elective specialty procedures. Often a patient's first-year budget is sufficient only for minor restorative and foundational care. If so, do not refer a patient to discuss specialty procedures she cannot afford. Instead, tell the patient that, at some point, she will be seen by a specialist who will help complete the lifetime strategy. When she asks how much the specialty fees will be, tell her they have already been estimated within the lifetime strategy. This is a wonderful strategy to eliminate the "sticker shock" patients experience when they speak to team specialists.

Time for the Referral

The time is right for the general dentist to refer the patient to the team specialist when:

- The patient's treatment plan cannot continue without specialty care.
- The patient is aware of the estimated fees and time in treatment for specialty care and it's within his budget.
- The patient has a solid relationship with the general dentist.

The referral process dialogue is important. Let's eavesdrop on a conversation between a general dentist and the patient. He's about to refer this patient to a specialist for dental implant placement. They're seated in the consultation area. Her chart sits closed in front of him and a telephone is on a table near where they are sitting.

"Mrs. Schartzer, do you remember when I told you some of your treatment would be completed by specialist?" Dr. Molzan, the general dentist, asks.

"Yes, I do, Dr. Molzan. You said that I needed dental implants and someone else would do that work."

"Let me tell you about who will be seeing you. Her name is Dr. Kristen Homoly. She's a gum and bone specialist and her office is just one block from here. We'll give you a map and it's easy to find. Dr. Homoly is one of the finest specialists in the area. I've been working with her for five years and our patients really enjoy her. She has advanced training in implant dentistry and patients come from all over the region to see her. Do you have any questions or comments about why you're seeing her?"

"Will I have the implants done on the first visit?"

"No. Dr. Homoly will examine you first, probably take a few x-rays, and then outline a plan of care for you. She'll communicate the plan to me also, so I'll know where you are in treatment every step of the way."

"How much will the implants cost?"

"The total fees for your implants have already been estimated within the treatment plan that I have done for you. I estimate Dr. Homoly's fees to be in the 6,000-dollar range. You'll pay those fees directly to her office and they will handle all of the

insurance work related to your care there. She has already seen your x-rays and we've talked about your case."

"Yes, I remember you telling me this. Plus you mentioned it in the letter I received from your office. When should I go to see Dr. Homoly?"

"Let me get her on the telephone right now." Dr. Molzan dials the specialist's office while the patient is present, so she can listen in. *"This is Dr. Molzan calling and I'm referring Mrs. Schartzer to Dr. Homoly for implant placement. Is Dr. Homoly available to come to the telephone?"*

"Dr. Homoly is with a patient right now, but I'll be glad to have her return your call. Can I give your patient appointment and referral information?" asks Ginger, the specialist's receptionist.

"Let me ask her," Dr. Molzan replies. *"Mrs. Schartzer, I have Ginger, Dr. Homoly's receptionist, on the line and she's available to schedule your appointment right now. Would you like to talk with her?"* Dr. Molzan hands the telephone to Mrs. Schartzer and she and Ginger discuss appointment procedures while the general dentist makes the referral entry in the patient's record.

Following this conversation, Mrs. Schartzer is brought to the front desk and is given referral information, including maps and introductory letters.

"You'll love Dr. Homoly," says Lily, Dr. Molzan's reception-ist. *"All our patients say the nicest things about her and she has a great staff there, too. Ginger is the receptionist there and we attend many continuing education programs together. You'll like her. I'll make sure they have all your x-rays and models that they'll need to plan your case."*

"Thank you so much. You've made this easy for me," Mrs. Schartzer says. She's smiling as she leaves.

Great Referrals

Let's analyze this dialogue and discover the components that make for great referrals.

A. The referral was not a surprise. Early in the relationship, when the dentist realized the patient would be treated within a team approach, the patient was informed. When it was time for the referral, there were no surprises or disappointments.

B. The dentist offered strong testimony for the credibility of the specialist. The staff was specific in its praise, citing the accomplishments and favorable history you've experienced while working with your specialist team member.

C. The staff was enthusiastic about the referral. Staff members' tone of voice and body language—attitude—communicate that they were happy the patient was taking the next step in treatment.

D. The patient was told what to expect at the first appointment with the team specialist. The staff removed as many unknowns as possible from the referral process.

E. The patient understood that the dentist would be in contact with the specialist and would monitor her treatment. She was given a sense of the dentist's continued involvement in her care.

F. The patient was reminded of the expected fees and time in treatment with the specialist. This probably required some "behind-the-scenes" work between the general dentist and the team specialist.

A major mistake within the team approach to case acceptance is to refer without informing the patient of expected fees.

G. The dentist made the telephone call to the team specialist's office in the presence of the patient. He showed the patient that this referral was so important to him that he was willing to handle it personally.

H. The patient made the referral appointment while still in the dentist's office (Do this whenever possible).

I. The patient was given maps to the team specialist's office and offered brochures on the planned specialty procedures.

J. The staff offered strong testimonial endorsement of the team specialist. Recommendations from staff members have a significant impact on the patient.

K. Later, the general dentist followed up by making sure the team specialist office knew his intended treatment plan, estimated fees, time in treatment, and necessary radiographs and study models.

Remember the distinction between teamwork and team harmony? How many aspects of a *great referral* relate to team harmony—attitude, good communication, collegiality? *Great referrals are 90 percent team harmony and 10 percent teamwork.*

Dr. Stuart Graves, an oral surgeon from Burke, Virginia, believes this kind of case acceptance process makes a big difference in the team approach to dentistry. *"I see more referrals—and better qualified referrals,"* he says, *"and the relationship between our staff and the referring office staff is much better because we're all on the same page. We've standardized our language so patients hear similar things in both offices. The concept of the dental budget is a major advantage to us. Patients know what our approximate fee is before they even come in. This saves time, not to mention headaches. We're doing more cases and bigger cases because of this process—it's as if I'm practicing in the same office as my referring doctor."*

In the Specialist's Office

At the patient's first appointment with the specialist, it should be obvious to the patient that:

- The specialist's office is aware of the patient's treatment plan.
- The team offices respect each other and enjoy working together.
- All diagnostic materials are present in the specialist's office.

Here's a sample dialogue that meets these criteria during the first few minutes of the patient's experience with the specialist.

"Mrs. Schartzer, I'm Dr. Kristen Homoly and we're pleased to have you here with us today. I've discussed your care with Dr. Molzan and I'm well aware of your treatment plan. You made a great decision when you chose Dr. Molzan as your dentist. He and I have treated patients together for years and I'm impressed with his thoroughness and skill.

"We've received your x-rays and study models from his office and today I will examine you and we'll talk about how we can best help you."

Case acceptance of the anticipated specialty procedures is predictable if all previous steps of the team approach to case acceptance have been accomplished. If the patient refuses specialty procedures, it's a direct result of poor patient preparation prior to the specialist case presentation. Here are some typical reasons patients reject specialty care:

- The patient doesn't understand why specialty procedures are required, and the general dentist assumes (hopes) the specialist will sell the case. Before the referral is made, the patient should know without a doubt that specialty procedures are required.
- Wide gaps exist in the technical knowledge about the dentistry planned by the respective teams. For example, in team treatment within implant dentistry, the general dentist doesn't understand the fundamentals of the surgical

diagnosis, implant placement, and healing, and the specialist doesn't understand the reconstructive and occlusal requirements. Each team doctor should be able to competently diagnose the respective team member's dentistry.

- The patient gets confused within the team approach. Patients become confused because the teams are confused. This occurs when the patient arrives at the specialist's office after there has been little discussion of the patient's treatment plan. It's not the patient's responsibility to make her team offices communicate. Team offices often spend more energy focusing on "getting their acts together" than they spend focusing on the patient.

It's insulting to patients that treating offices don't respect them enough to share information.

- The patient is surprised by the fees, financial arrangements, and insurance coverage. These issues are nearly always avoidable if both teams communicate to each other their financial policies. Always prepare patients for anticipated specialty fees whenever possible.
- The patient becomes discouraged because the specialist doesn't agree with or understand the general dentist's treatment plan. If the specialist doesn't agree with a treatment plan or recommends significantly more dentistry

than anticipated, the patient should not be the messenger who brings that "news" back to the general dentist. The specialist should tell the patient she will discuss her finding with the general dentist and together they will determine the best care. Never, ever use the patient as the bearer of bad news!

Case Discussion Letter and Consent

Each office must provide informed consent prior to starting treatment. The case discussion can be co-authored by each team dentist or each doctor can write separate letters.

Living Happily Ever After

Case acceptance for specialty procedures within the team approach is predictable when each office fulfills its role. When that happens, patients believe they are the center of attention, with each office focusing on them and following through on their commitments. When this occurs, they feel appreciated, important, and say yes to team treatment. Unlike battling married couples and their weary children, team treatment offices and their patients can learn to grow harmoniously, never regretting saying, "I do."

CHAPTER 18

Patients Are
Always Greener
On the **Other Side**
Of the
Fence

Converting Emergency and Recall Patients
to Complete Care Patients

I love hearing stories from dentists who have superstar celebrity patients. Think about it—someone has to treat Howard Stern. Chances are it's not you. You treat ordinary folks, you have a ton of recall patients, and you have more than your share of emergencies. Here are the facts: You'll be happier, do more of the dentistry you love, and make more money by treating your existing and emergency patients like celebrities than by going after high-profile new patients and focusing on diseases of the rich. Patients are always greener on the other side of the fence.

There are three ways to enter into the process of case acceptance for complete care: new patients, emergency patients, and re-care patients. The process I've described so far in this book focuses on new patients, but this represents only one way to bring patients into the fold.

Emergency Patients

Emergency patients can be a good source of complete care patients. Emergencies can be disruptive; however, when the emergency patient is a target patient, then it makes sense to process the emergency case as you would a new patient. Use your ability to identify and appoint target patients (CD-1) when you take the telephone call from the emergency patient. If you discover that he's a target patient, and if you have the opportunity to bring him in when you normally see new patients, you increase your chances of creating the right first impression on this patient.

For example, Tim calls your office with a broken front tooth. He's not a patient of record, and during the call you discover he's fifty-one, has missing teeth, and has heard good things about your office. You appoint him that afternoon and alert your staff that Tim is a target patient.

Tim is processed into your practice exactly as if he were a new patient. He's seen by the dentist first, a radiograph of the area is made, you do a simple initial examination to understand his disability. Because his concern is immediate and obvious, you treat his chief complaint. Only after he's pleased and comfortable do you offer the lifetime strategy for dental health, CD-2. This offer can be made by anyone in the office.

"Tim, I'm glad we were able to take care of you. Before you go, let me recommend that when you're ready, we can do a complete examination for you so we can prevent emergencies like this happening again. Have you ever thought about developing a lifetime strategy for dental health?" Review chapter 13 on CD-2 for the skills necessary to move forward from this point.

Expect the typical questions, resistance, and comments. However, if you use the information I've given you, you can easily manage this patient.

Re-care

Many general dentists' offices have multiple hygienists who see over sixty-four re-care patients a week, over 200 a month. Of the 200, is it not possible to convert one chief complaint patient to a complete care patient? I think it's possible. And do you know what one more complete care patient a month will do for your practice? Plenty. The secret to converting re-care patients to complete care is asking if they want to continue as a chief complaint patient or pursue a lifetime strategy—CD-2.

There's abundant opportunity in the re-care system to offer patients complete care.

Don't Look Under the Hood

At the re-care appointment, use your communications skills before your clinical skills. Let's say you take your car to a Sears service center, ask for an oil change, and do a little shopping while the work is being done. When you return to pick up your car, the service manager says you need new belts, hoses, and your master cylinder is leaking. What's your first thought? "Do I really need this work?"

Carolyn is in for her six-month recall. You clean her teeth, and when you're done, you tell her she needs two crowns and bleaching. What's her first thought? "Do I really need belts, hoses, and a master cylinder?"

What do these scenarios have in common? Recommendations were made only after you looked under the hood. This triggered suspicion, which translates to: "Do I really need this work?"

A strong and persuasive approach to offering a lifetime strategy for dental health is using your communication skills *before* your clinical skills.

Asking a patient if she'd like to talk about developing a lifetime strategy for dental health and appearance is an important question. Patients who think in terms of lifetime plans are more open to our suggestions. If we go into the recall appointment looking for dental problems, we teach patients to stay away or become suspicious. Have you ever heard a patient say, "You're not going to find anything wrong today, are you?"

Before the re-care patient is seated, study the record. Then think about the likely changes you could see in the patient's dental health. For example, Chester, your recall patient, is fifty-five and has many missing back teeth. The most likely changes in his mouth are going to be loose anterior teeth, tipping of posterior teeth, incisal edge wear, aesthetics, and worsening periodontal problems.

After Chester is seated and you've reviewed his medical history, start the CD-2 dialogue. *"Chester, I'm glad to clean your teeth today, but tell me, is this a good time for you to think about..."* and then recount what you believe will be the most obvious changes in his mouth. If you can tell him what his problems are before you've examined him, you increase the impact of your recommendations.

Let's take your car to Sears again. Instead of the mechanic recommending new belts, hoses, and a master cylinder after he's looked under the hood, what if he said: "Before we do your oil change, let me ask you a few questions. I'm familiar with your model car because we service them every day. This model tends to blow radiator hoses which can overheat your car and damage the fan and power steering belts. Have you had any problems with overheating or have you heard a squealing sound when you turn the steering wheel?" Does telling you about expected problems before he works on your car add credibility to his recommendations after he's looked under the hood? Yes, it does.

Our best recommendations are based on our experience, not stumbled across during an examination.

The best mechanics, dentists, and hygienists can see problems coming before we look under the hood. Ask patients if they'd like to talk about ways they can improve the appearance of, or replace, whiten, or seal their teeth. If you know that your patient has missing teeth or has teeth that would benefit from aesthetic dentistry, offer the chance to discuss it before you start your clinical procedures. Patients are tired after their appointments and may be out of time and energy to talk.

Kim, the hygiene assistant in the office of Drs. John and Julie Howard in Savannah, Georgia, has a wonderful way of introducing lifetime care. She says: *"Today, I'm glad to clean your teeth, or would you like the choice of talking about how we can..."* and she offers procedures that match patients' needs, such as bleaching, sealants, tooth replacements, and cosmetic care.

If the patient expresses interest in a lifetime strategy, then evaluate your time and the availability of the dentist. Ideally go right into the diagnostic appointment, renewing all diagnostic materials. After the diagnostic appointment, enter into CD-3, introducing the concept of the dental budget.

Dr. Jacques Doueck of Brooklyn, New York, talks about converting long-standing hygiene patients into complete care patients: *"Right after we finished our training with you we had an adult recall patient we have been seeing for years. She's had four partial dentures and is still not happy. Instead of cleaning her teeth, Emma, our hygienist, offered her a lifetime strategy. The patient jumped at the offer and we're now working her case up for fixed bridgework."*

Annual Plan

Another topic to introduce before starting clinical procedures is the annual plan for re-care. This is for patients who've just completed complex dentistry. The annual plan for re-care takes the boring "every six months" mentality out of re-care and elevates it.

Dr. Mark Davis of Clearwater, Florida, creates annual re-care plans for his patients. Dr. Davis says: *"The first year after treatment is complete, we watch patients carefully. We'll clean their teeth and adjust their occlusion on an as-needed basis. We include the first year re-care fee—bite adjustments, cleanings, products—in the total treatment fee. After the first year, patients usually qualify themselves to what re-care schedule most suits them. We dispense all the home care products they need for a year. This way they get what they need without product-centered discussions every time they're in."*

A good structure to follow when explaining the annual plan for re-care includes these elements: Describe what it is, why it's important, how and when you're going to do it, what it costs, and the next step.

For example, here's a sample of the way a hygienist can explain an annual plan:

"Devin, I recommend we create an annual plan to keep your mouth healthy. Dr. Davis has done beautiful dentistry for you and we're going to keep things healthy for you. During the next year we want to see you four to six times or as much as we need to. We'll be cleaning your teeth, keeping your gums healthy, and making minor adjustments in your bite. Also I'm going to give you everything you need to take care of your teeth and gums— a year's supply of toothbrushes, toothpaste, mouth rinses, disclosing tablets, floss, and an irrigation unit. There are no additional fees for your annual care plan. Next year we'll evaluate your progress and help you continue an annual plan to keep your mouth healthy. Let me explain how to use these products."

The emergency and re-care target patients are predictable sources of complete care patients when you process them as if they were new patients. Don't think of them as recall or emergency patients, think of them as complete care patients waiting to happen.

CHAPTER 19

Start Doing
The **Dentistry**
You **Love**

Finding Target Patients

Case acceptance for complete dentistry and marketing are joined at the hip, and it's tough to advance one without the other. Complete care patients don't parade through your office; you must attract them. Internal marketing is a good start but isn't enough. Although patients may tell you that they have the best intentions of referring their friends and relatives, they have more to do than make your life easy. If you wait for target patients to find you, you'll have skinny kids.

For twenty-five years I've watched dentists flock like geese to continuing education courses. They absorb hundreds of hours of advanced clinical techniques, only to lay eggs when they try to implement what they learned.

Clinical skills, it turns out, are more easily learned than they are put to use. And this creates a problem of "excess capacity," which in this context means knowing much more than you actually have the opportunity to do. Excess capacity over time leads to frustration, low profitability, and nagging doubts. You're all dressed up with no place to go.

Jerry is a highly educated general dentist who has hundreds of hours of continuing education in restorative dentistry. He feels great about his clinical skills and receives offers to lecture to study clubs and associations. Jerry asked me to help him with his practice and his speaking career.

"I almost feel like a fake," Jerry said. "Here I have offers to talk to groups and yet I'm having problems getting enough big cases to do myself."

"So, is it that you don't have enough new patients, or the ones you have don't accept care?" I asked.

"Both," said Jerry.

"How do you market your practice?"

Jerry winced. "I don't see advertising in our town. I don't want to spread my name all over the place. Chiropractors and podiatrists do that and I hate it."

"What is it that you hate about it?"

"They look cheap and needy," Jerry said. "Listen, I know they provide some good things. I go to the chiropractor once a month for my neck and back and he's a great guy. But the advertisements, with the drawings of spinal cords and their pictures, is just too much for me."

Like many dentists, Jerry is looking for the ways to attract target patients to his office and have them accept care. And, like many dentists, Jerry is not clear what marketing really is and how to make it happen for him.

What Makes Me the Expert?

In 1979 when it became legal and ethical, I hired a public relations firm to market my practice of implant and restorative dentistry. I aggressively marketed my practice for twenty years. I learned what worked and what didn't. I advertised in newspapers, magazines, radio, television, and direct mail. I appeared on every television talk show in North and South Carolina as well as many radio talk shows. I was featured in *Life* magazine and spoke to hundreds of civic groups and local, state, regional, and national dental associations. I have served on the public relations committee for the American Academy of Implant Dentistry for many years and was its chairperson at one point. In 1986 I started Homoly Marketing Group, which specializes in attracting target patients to high-end restorative practices and during that time have served several hundred clients. My experience with marketing professional dental services is extensive and hands-on.

You must understand the following four principles of marketing:

1. Market your practice only after you have solid operational systems. Marketing a practice with weak systems creates stress and leads to mistakes, low returns, and hair loss.

2. Market your practice only after you've learned to sell dentistry. If you don't, you'll hear no more often, have more stress, and make less money.

3. Once you start marketing, never quit. Marketing takes time and most dentists quit long before they see results.

4. Marketing is leadership. It's not about you, it's about getting the good news of contemporary dentistry to the public. Focus on targeting the right message to the right people so they have the best opportunity to access care. Do this well and you'll prosper.

Marketing Ins and Outs

From the consumer's point of view, dentistry has two components: dentistry and the dentist. Before a patient says yes to your treatment recommendations, she needs to be sold twice, once on the concept of the dentistry and again on the dentist who'll do it. One is a conceptual sell, the other is a relationship sell.

The greatest leverage in conceptual selling is promoting target dentistry outside your office. The best way to build the relationships is to promote yourself inside your office. Promote the dentistry outside, yourself inside.

A solid strategy about marketing is to promote target dentistry outside your practice (the "Outs"), and promote yourself inside the practice (the "Ins").

Many dentists make the mistake of doing the reverse; they promote themselves outside, and their dentistry inside. When they promote themselves outside the office, it reeks of self-centeredness. When they promote their dentistry inside the office, they can come across tooth-centered.

Social Proof

To attract target patients —cosmetic, implant, restorative, and so forth—you must convince the public that target dentistry in general is a good thing. You do this by creating something called "social proof." One of the ways that individuals decide what is correct is to see what other people are doing. The greater number of people who find an idea correct, the more the idea will *be* correct. Social proof is most commonly built by the media, through "paid media" (generally advertising) and through "earned media," which are stories about the target dentistry in question.

Cigarette smoking is a good example of the power of social proof. Not too long ago, most Americans smoked cigarettes, and even those who didn't kept ashtrays on hand so their guests would feel free to light up. Now, just try to find an ashtray in a nonsmoker's home. In fact, many smokers won't indulge in their own homes! Media reports had a direct impact on these changes; they created social proof of the dangers of smoking.

Advertising and publicity are the best ways to reach the public with the concept of target dentistry and building social proof. The challenge is how to do both well and stay within your budget.

Figure Out Your Budget

The greatest effect on your budget is location. When it comes to conceptual selling, suburban and rural dentists have a big advantage over the urban dentist. The costs associated with advertising and publicity in rural and suburban areas are much less than in the big cities. Additionally, small-town and suburban dentists pay less for rent and labor costs, giving them more money to use in a marketing budget. Although patient fees are higher in urban areas, they generally are not so high that they offset the additional costs of marketing.

I'm always amused when I hear a dentist boast, "I have a million dollar practice and I did it all in a small town!" I think, "Of course you did it in a small town, that's the easiest place to do it—wages are low, ad rates are cheap, facility costs are minor. Try doing it in a large northern city where you'll bust your chops on managed care, stiff competition, high salaries and facility costs, and prima donna patients."

Regardless of how creative your advertising looks and how wealthy and cosmopolitan your area is, if you don't have the budget to reach your target market with enough frequency to build awareness, you lose.

The Best Bang for the Buck

Print (newspapers, direct mail, magazines) and broadcast (television and radio) media are the primary vehicles for advertising and publicity. Based on twenty-five years of experience working with hundreds of clients nationwide, the best dollar-for-dollar return in marketing for most dental practices is newspaper advertising and publicity. The best one-two punch for building social proof is to combine advertising and publicity, i.e., having a feature article written about target dentistry and having an advertisement in the same issue.

The next best return in print is publicity, i.e., an article written about dentistry in which you are included as an expert source. Studies have shown that people are ten to thirteen times more likely to believe articles in the newspaper than other advertisements of equal size. Articles have shelf life. People read them, cut them out, and put them in a drawer. When they're ready for treatment, they find the article, call your office and show up, sometimes years later, with your yellowed article in hand. The big disadvantage of newspaper publicity is that it's hard to land an article, and if you do, don't expect to do another for years to come. Although the credibility of a newspaper article is sky high, the frequency is very low.

For most dentists, newspaper print advertising is the most doable and profitable tool for building social proof. Here, frequency is key. Run your advertisements for at least thirteen-week intervals, twice a year. Pitch the deepest disability or the greatest benefit you can offer in your headline. Your name (or practice name) is not a headline and doesn't do anything to build social proof. Have your advertisements designed by professionals. Position them in the newspaper sections your target patients are most likely to read (food, travel, finance, and obituaries).

Broadcast media generally reach more people than print media do. For most dentists, the best buy in broadcast is network television. The response time in television is much shorter than for print material. The disadvantages of television include cost and lack of shelf life; viewers can't keep a television ad in their home-office drawer. A good way to reduce your costs and extend the shelf life of television advertising is to combine your advertising dollars with other dentists who have similar goals and cooperatively market your practices.

The concept of cooperative marketing is growing in popularity in dentistry, and the history and techniques of cooperative marketing are evolving. Cooperative marketing, whether in print or broadcast, is an excellent answer to the problem of the costs and risks associated with building social proof that contemporary dentistry is good news. No method is perfect, and I have had good and bad results in cooperative marketing efforts.

Advertising and publicity take considerable time and experience, and dentists don't have much of either one. So, just as you would hire an accountant or attorney, use professionals to help you design and implement your marketing plans.

The Ins of Marketing

I spent a few days in Dr. Larry's office. He was having trouble selling big cases. Carolyn, his top chair-side assistant, put her finger right on the problem. "Dr. Larry is a wonderful dentist. I wouldn't work for anyone else. But he just doesn't come across as enthusiastic to the patients about dentistry as I know he really is. And he gives them so much technical detail, they get confused and end up asking me what he said and what they should do."

Larry's problems were good ones—he had plenty of target patients. He and his partner had created social proof in their community for the value of target dentistry. *His problem was that he couldn't shut up long enough for them to say yes.*

Once the social proof is created, patients will come looking for you. And that's when relationship selling begins. Many dentists make a mistake in thinking they need to sell the dentistry in detailed technical terms.

Most patients need to know more about you than they need to know about the technical aspects of care.

The fact that patients are in your office is evidence that they have experienced adequate social proof—ads, publicity, referrals—that target dentistry may be right for them. Now it's time for them to decide if you're the dentist to do it. You can help them decide in your favor by building a personal relationship based on issues we've already discussed:

- Philosophy: Focus on target patients, build value early, know the difference between quality and suitability, understand the difference between dental IQ and readiness.
- Attitude, connection, disclosure, and visual language

- The Spectrum of Appeal
- StorySelling
- The Five Critical Dialogues

How Not to Market

Starting in the mid-'80s I taught dentists how to market their practices. I wrote a manual, recorded audiotapes, and gave hands-on workshops. Looking back, I'm convinced marketing your practice yourself is the worst way to accomplish your goals. Worse yet is giving the marketing duties to a staff member.

Most staff members have no marketing experience, don't have time, and don't love it.

Find a small local advertising or public relations firm to help you. I know several. If you need one, call me.

The Boutique Practice

Many general dentists talk about a boutique practice, one that caters only to a narrow range of procedures and is known as a niche practice. At the time of this writing, mid-2000, the niche of the day is cosmetic dentistry. In the 1980s and 1990s it was TMJ or implants, and before then it was cast gold restorations.

I believe, for most general practitioners, that developing a niche practice for cosmetic, implant, or TMJ, and so forth, is a mistake. Here's why. Most cosmetic, implant, TMJ, and restorative work is generated out of the general practice. If you chase off your general practice because you're ravenous for niche care, you'll have less to do, and less money to work with.

It's much smarter to do what is necessary to keep your general practice healthy and find an associate or partner to help you run it. Then within the general practice build your portion to be 25 to 40 percent target patients. If you try to build an exclusive practice with only target patients, you'll be disappointed. Most GPs will end up with the same problems that specialists have today. Most specialists would love to be associated with a big general practice (with someone else running it), referring them the target care. You already have that now, so why throw it away?

You might say, "Yeah, how about the GPs who have built specialty practices with target patients? If they can do it, so can I."

It's true that a few GPs have built the "niche" practice, myself included. However, "niching" your practice is like adhering to practice philosophy; too much rigidity will hurt you. Looking back on my experience and seeing where many niche practitioners are today, here are some reasons to not go overboard in limiting your general practice:

- Niche practices are hard to sell. How many dentists do you know who would buy a practice exclusive to implant and restorative practice?
- Niche practitioners rely heavily on patient referrals and/or external marketing. How many general practitioners are anxious to refer cosmetic or implant dentistry to another general practitioner colleague?

- Niche practices must succeed outside the dental insurance industry. Although this may sound inviting, unless you have exemplary people skills, dynamite marketing, and a great practice location, kicking dental insurance out the door is easier said than done.
- Most niche practitioners I know have given 200 percent to their practices, which is good for the practice but plays like hell at home. The satisfaction of treating only target patients often is offset by the struggle necessary to generate them. Often these struggles are projected onto home life, and nothing will cripple your practice more than an unsuccessful life at home.

The Spectrum of Appeal

Figure 1 shows the relationship between differentiating your dentistry and yourself. When practicing low-fee tooth dentistry, the dentistry is differentiated—price, office hours, convenience, insurance, speed of delivery, and options. These are generally blue spectrum characteristics.

When practicing complete dentistry, it is the dentist who is differentiated by character, personality, and reputation. These are red spectrum characteristics. When the fees are high, patients look beyond the dentistry and look more carefully at the dentist.

Patients know that dentistry can fail, whether it's high- or low-fee. When low-fee tooth dentistry fails, it is a simple matter of a technical repair. When complete dentistry fails, it is the dentist's character, personality, or reputation that enables the technical repair.

FIGURE 1: Differentiate your dentistry and yourself.

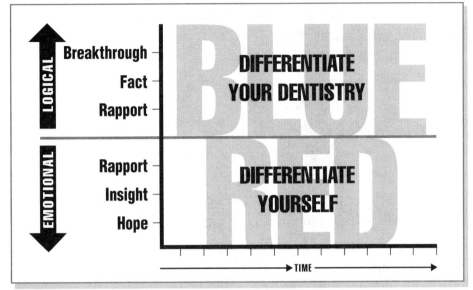

It is this promise of a dentist's character, personality, and reputation that the patients buy when they accept complete care.

When you differentiate your practice based on the dentistry, a blue spectrum approach, then competition on price, quality, location, and convenience can occur. When you differentiate your practice based on your character and personality, a red spectrum approach, no one can compete with you on that basis. No one can be you.

The best marketing strategy is to differentiate your dentistry in the blue spectrum and differentiate yourself in the red.

Take Action

Here's how to start the marketing process:

- Find an experienced marketing/promotional specialist. Look for a small agency that will value your account and give it the attention it needs. Large agencies tend to underserve and overcharge small accounts such as those dentists typically bring.
- Collect testimonials from happy patients. These testimonials endorse the process of dentistry. They can be used to build social proof in advertising and publicity and they make great stories when building relationships.
- Determine your marketing budget. Budgets can vary from 4 percent to 10 percent of gross collections, depending on the impact and response rate you want.
- Spend your budget from the inside out. First, develop in-office relationship tools, such as personal and staff communication/relationship skills, telephone skills, and facility improvements. Then develop outside promotional tools.

When you begin a promotion plan, you will need to consider your preferred or target market. In the next chapter, you'll learn why youth isn't all it's cracked up to be.

CHAPTER 20

Dentures
Can Make Your
Restorative
Practice Click

Finding Older Patients

For most general dentists, making a denture is a giant step backward, back to dental school, that is, and the nightmare denture patient from hell. It seems "cool" to have upscale, young, articulate patients than the older crowd. But your yuppie patients are "spent out." As a group, they have great teeth, and don't have one-tenth the dentistry in their mouths that you need to make a living. If you want to do more complete dentistry, you need to see more patients with fewer teeth!

Dr. Tom was having trouble with dentures. Not his dentures—Tom has a full set of fine teeth. He was having trouble with his *patients'* dentures or, more specifically, the lack thereof. "I just don't see many patients who need rehabilitations," Tom told me after my workshop on complete dentistry. "I can't sell them if they don't walk in the door."

Tom has a busy general practice. He does a large amount of cosmetic dentistry and traditional fixed prosthetics, restoring one to three teeth at a time. Despite his success he wants to expand his practice into rehabilitative care, but he seems to be stuck doing smaller cases.

"How may full dentures did you make last year?" I asked.

"Very few, probably less than five."

"Your problem is that you have too many patients with teeth in your practice," I told him. "Too many teeth can interfere with practice growth." Tom laughed but stopped after he realized I wasn't kidding.

"I suspect most of your patients are your age, plus or minus five years, which makes them between twenty-five and thirty-five. The people in your circle of influence, your friends, family, and acquaintances, are predominately under forty years old. How many people in your circle of influence wear dentures?"

"None of my friends do. A few of my relatives do, but they're not patients in my practice," he replied.

"Tom, if you want to do more rehabilitative care you must do two things: First, you need to age your patient base by one or two decades," I said. "Next, you need to attract the partially and fully edentulous patient to your practice. It's like we're in the car repair business. Would we do more work by focusing on new cars or old cars? Old cars. Tom, you need more 'old cars' in your practice."

To reinforce this message, consider the "numbers." Bob Ganley, president of Ivoclar North America, reminds us that:

- People age fifty and older spend $525 billion annually on health care.
- People fifty and older control half of this country's disposable income and 75 percent of the financial assets.
- The sixty-five-plus age group is the fastest growing demographic in North America and will double by the year 2030.
- Twelve million new dentures are made every year.
- It's estimated that 32 million Americans are edentulous and of this population, 75 percent have old dentures that need to be replaced.

Like many dentists, Tom is caught in the generation gap, the gap between him and the patients he wants to treat. Tom's generation and that of most of his patients are too young to support a rehabilitative dentistry practice.

Attracting Older Patients

A predictable way to attract patients who are at least fifty years old and need complex restorative care is to market to the full denture patient. There are some solid reasons that marketing to full denture patients is great for your restorative practice.

First, when you market to fully edentulous patients, they tend to respond well to your messages. For most patients, total edentulism is the deepest and most devastating dental disability.

Unlike a thirty-year-old with a missing molar, the older totally edentulous patient is more profoundly affected by her dental condition. It affects her health, appearance, and self-confidence. Full denture patients are aware of the problem every moment. Because they are aware of their profound disability, they respond well to your marketing messages.

Second, marketing to full denture patients will attract a wide variety of dentistry, including individuals who want cosmetic care, dental implants, crown and bridge, periodontics, and oral surgery. These patients want to look better, feel better, and speak better. I marketed to the fully edentulous patient for twenty years and my primary purpose was to treat dental implant patients. In the process of attracting the fully edentulous patient, I also attracted patients who needed cosmetic care and crown and bridge, which kept my full-time associate busy and happy.

Third, older patients are willing to spend money to improve their dental health. *A full denture is the mark of old age.* Many older patients have the money and are willing to spend what it takes to postpone the emotional tolls of the aging process.

Push and Pull

The first rule when marketing dentures is appealing to the emotions, the red spectrum, within the target market of men and women. Two components stand out within the emotional profile of this target market: *things they want more of, and things they want less of.* People in this group are pulled toward things that they want more of and they push away things they want less of. Smart marketing of dentures does both; smart marketing pulls patients toward what they want and pushes them away from what they don't want.

The leading pull for most women is aesthetics, and for most men it's function. Women are pulled toward better face and lip support, whiter teeth, more natural denture base shades, and more display of teeth when talking and smiling. Men are pulled toward being able to chew steak, eat corn on the cob, hold a pipe between their teeth, and speak more clearly.

The push, what denture patients want less of, is the opposite of the pull. For women the push is looking old; short, dull teeth; cheap-looking teeth; and facial creases. A phenomenally strong *push* for women is being seen without their dentures. The push for men is soft diets, inconvenience, and slurred speech.

Here are some steps to follow for attracting denture patients:

- Upgrade your denture clinical techniques.
- Send direct mail to your patients who are over forty-five years old, highlighting your new and improved denture services.
- Speak to civic and church groups about the miracles of modern dentistry.
- Host public seminars about denture, implant, and cosmetic dentistry.
- Team up with colleagues who share your vision and cooperatively advertise to attract the older patient.

Get good and fast at dentures and you'll do more cosmetic and restorative dentistry. Bring older patients into your practice and increase your opportunities to offer complete dentistry.

CHAPTER 21

Everyone **Wants to Go to Heaven,** No One Wants to **Die**

Asking for Patient Referrals

I've discovered a predictable way to make dentists squirm. I just bring up the topic of asking patients for referrals. All dentists want patient referrals, but most dentists and staff members hate asking for them. However, if you want referrals, learn how to ask. Everyone wants to go to heaven; no one wants to die.

Asking for referrals is not a topic that comes up naturally in conversations with patients. Consequently, to many of us, it sounds like begging. Brian, a client on the West Coast, summed up this attitude when he said, "I'm uncomfortable asking my patients for referrals. I don't know what to say, or how to say it, and I don't want to sound as if I need patients."

Patient referrals are an obstacle for most of us. But like many obstacles we face, this one contains opportunity that is knocking and wants to come out and greet you. If you and your staff agree with Brian then *quit asking for referrals and start recommending them.* Here's how.

Be aware that the patient with chronic inflammatory and degenerative dental diseases, and partial and total edentulism, often suffers from other chronic diseases, particularly cardiovascular disease and diabetes. In February 1998 *USA Today* reported that gum disease is linked to heart disease. The article was based on research done at the University of Minnesota and linked systemic diseases such as cardiovascular disease, diabetes, and premature birth to periodontal disease. More recently, conflicting research challenged earlier conclusions. I'm sure additional research will follow. The point is that we know that oral health and general systemic health are linked. This link between poor oral health and overall health creates the opportunity to quit asking for referrals and start recommending them.

This link between poor oral health and poor overall health creates the opportunity to quit asking for referrals and start recommending them.

Begin to see the medical history as more than a clinical tool. The medical history, when combined with a patient interview, opens doors to referrals because it gives insights into family history. For example, your new patient is fifty-seven years old, has a history of heart disease, and has moderate periodontal disease. Chances are good that he has family members or relatives with a similar medical and dental history. After building a relationship with this patient, you can have the following dialogue:

"Mr. Chambers, are you aware that gum disease might aggravate heart disease?"

"No, doctor, I didn't know that."

"Yes, it might, and the problem is that patients may not realize they have gum disease. You can have it and not know it, and if you have a history of heart problems, gum disease can aggravate your condition. Do you have any family members or relatives with heart disease?"

"As a matter of fact I do. Both of my brothers have heart problems."

"Are your brothers being seen by a dentist regularly to monitor their gum health?"

"I don't think so. You know, nobody likes going to the dentist."

"Here's my recommendation. Have your brothers call this office and we'll do a gum health screening examination for them. You'll be doing them a big favor if they have gum disease but don't know it."

The medical history represents a tremendous opportunity as a referral tool, but it is unused and dormant in most dental offices. However, the advantages to this process are numerous. The recommendation for referral is much higher on the therapeutic playing field than are personal appeals. From my experience as a dental team trainer I have learned that staff and dentists are much more comfortable and skilled talking about issues related to treatment. Moreover, by using a therapeutic approach to recommending referrals, we offer patients something of great value in return for their referral. We offer them the opportunity to help people they love, which beats the traditional token flowers and thank-you cards for referrals.

Recommending a referral based on preventative issues is a much stronger appeal to the patient than the traditional "Send me your friends" approach.

If you're interested in recommending referrals, here are some suggestions:

- Read the studies linking periodontal disease to systemic health.

- Practice recommending referrals in role-play situations with your staff. Everyone on your team should be comfortable with the language of referrals and be able to use it effectively.
- Alert your local medical society. Offer an article on pertinent issues for its newsletter or speak to the group at a medical society meeting.

The opportunity for more consistent patient referrals using a therapeutic approach to recommending referrals is enormous. By finding important, urgent, and valid reasons for patients to refer others to you, you'll soon stop asking for referrals and begin recommending them.

Asking for Referrals

I feel strongly about asking for referrals and believe it's important that you become good at it. The skills in asking for referrals transcend dentistry. No matter what business you're in, asking for referrals is crucial. When my staff members moaned and groaned about the need to practice asking for referrals I'd tell them—in a good-natured way, of course—that they could either become good at it now or at their next job! So, to generate patient referrals, do the following:

- Ask early.
- Ask often.
- Ask everyone.
- Give patients a reason to refer.
- Have the right tools.
- Say thank you.

Ask Early

Ask patients for referrals early in your relationship. Review chapter 8 on value. *Patients are often more "jazzed" about getting their teeth fixed before the treatment begins because they are starting a process linked with self-esteem and in some cases, a "new start."* Ask for referrals when patients are fully involved with the process. If you wait until the end of treatment to ask, patients are relieved to be finished with the process and are no longer as emotionally involved.

Ask Often

Most of my dentist clients tell me they experience the highest level of referral activity while the patient is in treatment. If you're doing multiple units of cosmetic care, you'll have several appointments, hence opportunities, to ask. Think what only one referral from each of your patients would mean to your practice.

Ask Everyone

Asking for referrals is not just for patients who've completed care. Ask recall patients, emergency patients, vendors, and friends. I'm amazed at how the real estate industry works. My wife Carolyn sells residential real estate and I've seen how effectively she asks for referrals from her circle of influence. She doesn't push people, but she reminds them of her business by telling stories about houses she's sold, listed, or people she's worked with. She's in the top 4 percent of residential salespeople in the country. She asks for referrals. So should you.

Give Patients a Reason

As previously discussed, using the medical history is an excellent way to inspire referrals. Asking patients for referrals without giving a reason is weak and most dentists and staff don't like doing it. Look for a reason.

For example, if you're treating a woman for periodontal disease it's likely that periodontal disease exists in her husband and it contributes to her condition, too.

Have the Right Tools

Have the right tools for referrals; make it easy for people to refer to you. Use brochures, e-mail, websites, and after-hours information on recorded telephone messages. Full-face photographs with testimonial letters on the wall of your consultation room are powerful referral tools because of the strong human-interest stories attached to those photographs. These photos and letters encourage patients to tell stories about your practice. We call patient referrals word-of-mouth promotion. But it's not the word that generates referrals, it's the stories.

Say Thank You

People love recognition. If someone does something nice for you, be quick to say thank you. A thank you delivered face-to-face with a smile and a twinkle in your eye does wonders for relationships.

When You're Asked for a Referral

When you're asked for a referral from another businessperson, do it, and then ask for a referral in return. Smart businesspeople network with each other and help build each other's businesses.

When You're Asked by a Patient for a Reference

When a patient asks you for a reference, provide it, and then ask if he'd be willing to talk to people about the care he's received from you. For example, your new patient Clark asks, "Do you have any patients I can talk to about their cosmetic dentistry?"

"Clark, I have many and Ginger at the front desk can give you their names and numbers. I'm sure you'll like what you hear and when we're done with your care, would you be willing to talk to people about your experience?"

Complete dentistry lends itself to patient referrals because patients are in treatment longer, they have significant emotional concerns, and their level of commitment is high. Every patient will not refer others, no matter what you do. But what if you asked the right patient at the right time for a referral?

What would your practice be like if you could get just one complete care-patient referral a month? Try doing what this chapter suggests and be prepared to find out.

CHAPTER 22

Mars and Venus
In the
Dental
Office

---

*"**Mars and Venus in the Dental Office** helps you take a giant step towards building successful relationships with patients and staff members. In my video presentation and article with Dr. Paul Homoly you will see how you can easily adapt the concepts of **Men Are from Mars, Women Are from Venus** to the unique work environment of Dentistry."*

John Gray, Ph.D., Author of
Men Are from Mars, Women Are from Venus

The Mars/Venus concepts are broad patterns of behavior observed from over twenty years of experience by John Gray and others. Dr. Gray's work attempts to identify the differences between men and women, but are not intended to stereotype the behavior of the sexes. Many men have Venusian characteristics; many women, especially in the workplace, display Martian characteristics. He offers strategies that help us understand and appreciate our differences, which give us paths to follow to create harmony between men and women. Harmony is the lifeblood of case acceptance for complete dentistry.

In the fall 1997, my wife and I attended the Mars/Venus Institute in Mill Valley, California. We were trained by John Gray, Ph.D., and his staff to facilitate Mars/Venus workshops for married couples and singles. During our training, I approached John with some ideas for articles and courses on relationship issues in the dental office. He agreed with my vision and supports my effort to bring Mars/Venus concepts to dentistry. You'll find that after you become familiar with John Gray's work, you'll see many applications for it in dentistry and, in particular, case acceptance for complete dentistry.

Who's the Problem

At dinner one evening my client, Dr. Baker, shook his head and confessed, "It's a love-hate relationship between my staff and me. I can't get my staff to settle in and work like a team. The harder I try, the worse it gets. It's hard working with all women."

"What's the problem?" I asked.

"It's not what's the problem, it's who's the problem," he said.

"We've got a great office, but it seems like someone's always crabbing about something. It wears me out. And half the time I don't understand what they're complaining about."

"Do they know what's causing their problems?" I asked.

"Listen, they're supposed to know. That's why I pay them," he barked.

Can you identify with Dr. Baker's frustration? If so, then John Gray has an important book for you: *Men Are from Mars, Women Are from Venus*. Learning skills for dealing with the opposite sex are emotional intelligence skills, and although his book is intended to be a guide for married men and women, its principles apply directly to the men and women of dentistry. Here's how.

Mars and Venus

Imagine that men are from Mars and women are from Venus. On their respective planets, Martians and Venusians behaved and communicated quite differently. Achievement, competence, power, and efficiency motivated Martians. Venusians valued love, communication, and the quality of their relationships. Martians prided themselves on doing things all by themselves. For Venusians, it was a great sign of love to offer help to another Venusian without being asked.

And as legend has it, Martians and Venusians came to Earth to live together. And yes, they built dental offices, and together Martians and Venusians offered their patients a marvelous mixture of competency, efficiency, results, love, communication, beauty, and quality relationships. Martians and Venusians combined the best of their values to create heavenly dental practices.

And because they knew they were from different planets, they recognized and appreciated their differences. For example, on Mars when a Martian dentist was stressed, he'd go into his private office cave and silently think his problem through. At first this distressed the Venusian assistants because on Venus, when a Venusian had a problem, her friends would instinctively gather around her and they'd talk about it, which made them feel better. So on Earth, when the Martian dentist would go to his cave, their instincts were to draw him out and convene a staff meeting to discuss things. But the Martian dentist assured his Venusian assistants that a meeting was not necessary. He was happy to solve his problems alone. So the Venusians went about their tasks cheerfully chatting among themselves. And when he came out to treat his next patient, everything was just fine.

(Important note: Many excellent dentists were also Venusians!)

Martian dentists also realized that their assistants had needs quite different from their own. At the end of a long day of treating patients, an assistant would talk to her Martian dentist about how long and tiring the day was. She would talk about each aspect of the day's schedule, reliving the day's events, expressing how she felt. At first the Martian dentist thought he should try to solve her problems by offering solutions, thus trying to minimize her problems. After all, his job was to solve problems. But, the Venusian assistants told him it was not necessary for him to offer solutions and it was important that he not tell them or imply that their feelings were wrong. The Venusians just wanted to be heard and understood. That made them feel better and relieved their sense of being overwhelmed.

Because he knew they were from different planets, it was easy for him to listen and not offer solutions or make them wrong for feeling overwhelmed.

However, one night in their sleep, Martians and Venusians experienced selective amnesia and they forgot one very important thing: *They were from different planets.* They lost the awareness that they were supposed to be different. And the next day and every day since, Martians and Venusians in the dental office have been struggling to get along. It got so bad that an entire dental industry—practice management—sprang up over night.

Practice management consultants swarmed over dentistry trying to put out the fires between dentists and assistants. Their advice included complex incentive systems, personality profiles, and hammering the importance of staff meetings. Martian consultants invalidated Venusian emotions, while Venusian consultants tried to "fix" the Martians. Nothing worked consistently and *to this day the number one complaint Martians and Venusians in dentistry have is about each other.*

Could there be something our profession has overlooked, perhaps a principle of management that is fundamental to all practice management models? According to John Gray, there is. What we've overlooked is that the men and women of dentistry are supposed to be different. It's unrealistic to apply rigid practice management models that lump men and women together.

Men and women differ significantly in the following areas:
- The ways they manage stress
- What motivates them
- The way they communicate
- Their emotional cycles
- Their emotional needs
- What pleases them
- The way they ask for support

Cookie-Cutters

Look at the above list and tell me how the men and women of dentistry can prosper when the practice management model they follow does not recognize and adjust for fundamental gender differences. Many dental-practice management models ignore gender differences. They copy management models from other industries such as manufacturing, fast food, hotels, and sales and rubber-stamp them onto dentistry.

Years ago my staff and I attended a high-dollar, yearlong management program for dental offices. Like a cookie-cutter, it stamped out its rigid recommendations. I ended up frustrated and my staff was unhappy. Looking back on that experience, I understand why. It sought to standardize our behavior and attempted to create single-file solutions. Additionally, it failed to distinguish that men and women need different paths to reach the common practice goals.

Men and women of dentistry perform and succeed for their own reasons. Recognizing and appreciating our differences, not struggling against or being punished for our differences, is the key to practice harmony. Let's look at a few examples.

Dr. Davis is a master reconstruction dentist. His work is very demanding. By the end of the day he is physically and emotionally drained. When the last patient leaves, he goes into his office and flips through a few journals and without a word to anyone he disappears out the back door. His staff members are exhausted, too. And when they see him leave without a word to anyone they think something is wrong. They worry about his behavior: "Is he mad at us?" "Did we do something wrong?" "Is he going to fire us?" They become suspicious about what he may be thinking and assume the worst. Staff morale suffers and by the end of every week, the stress is suffocating. Everyone thinks something is terribly wrong.

The fact is, nothing is wrong. A Mars/Venus consultant would explain that it's normal for a Martian dentist to withdraw when stressed. Dr. Davis appreciates and respects his staff but lacks the capacity to express his feelings when stressed. Withdrawal is his coping mechanism and the staff should not interpret his withdrawal as a negative action. By recognizing and appreciating his need to withdraw, the staff will not feel threatened by his behavior. Dr. Davis should reassure his staff that there is nothing to worry about when he slips out the back door at the end of the day. Now the staffers can use their energy helping each other without fearing for their jobs.

Here's another example. Dr. Allen is exhausted by the constant breakdown in staff performance. Things will be going along fine, then staff issues will pop up and create havoc. The clinical staff will complain about the receptionist, and the office manger will start a war with the scheduler. Dr. Allen will convene a staff meeting, bring in a consultant, lay down the law, and things seem to settle down. Two weeks later, problems reappear. To him it seems impossible to level out the emotions and performance of his staff. He wants consistency and worries that something is wrong with his leadership.

There is nothing wrong with Dr. Allen's leadership. A Mars/Venus consultant would explain to him that the emotions and behavior of his Venusian staff will perpetually rise and fall like the waves in the ocean. You see, on Venus it's common knowledge that Venusians may suddenly experience a host of unexplained emotions. They may spontaneously feel hopeless and unsupported. But soon after they reach an emotional bottom, they can rise up and begin to radiate support to all. A Martian dentist will burn out trying to enforce an office environment based on even, level emotions. Instead, he should recognize and appreciate that from time to time, emotional waves will rise and crash around him. Smart leadership means not trying to calm the waves or get caught up in them.

Smart leadership means supporting, not struggling with, emotional issues.

Patient management is strongly influenced by Mars/Venus principles. Dr. Green prides himself on staying on schedule and his staff knows that running late is his pet peeve. Mrs. Chambers, his patient, is seated for her initial examination. As he is about to start, his chair-side assistant Lisa says, "Excuse me for a second, I've got to get one thing." Then she hops out of her chair. She returns in a minute, which seems like an eternity to Dr. Green. In a disapproving tone of voice he says, "Lisa, have the room set up on time, every time. Understood?"

What Mrs. Chambers, his patient, understands is that Dr. Green is capable of talking to her in the same disapproving tone. What's worse is that the trust Dr. Green seeks most from his patients is lost. A Mars/Venus consultant would tell Dr. Green that the way he treats the women around him signals to many of his Venusian patients the way he is capable of treating them. Whereas a Martian patient may appreciate Dr. Green's directness and punctuality, a Venusian patient may see it as a threat to her.

No woman likes to see another woman mistreated.

Mars and Venus principles influence case acceptance of complete dentistry. It's Thursday afternoon and it's been a tough week. So far today a few crowns didn't seat, collections for the month are way off, and the new patient, Mrs. McBucks, is thirty minutes late. Dr. Martian and his staff are feeling the stress from all the normal but unacceptable circumstances of practicing dentistry.

Mrs. McBucks has also had a tough day. She's worried for weeks about this appointment. She has some friends who had dental work that looked bad, which made her so anxious she woke up with a headache. Then she got lost driving into the city to find the dental office. For her, today seems like one of those days. The dentist, his staff, and the female patient are all under stress.

When stressed dentists, assistants, and patients have to interact, and the way they treat each other is often not what any of them need to relieve their stress. In particular, *the stressed male dentist and the stressed female patient can be like oil and water.*

What does the stressed female patient naturally want to do? She wants to talk about her dental problems. She expects the dentist will want to hear all the details from her decades of dental problems, previous dentists, poor dental experiences, what her friends say about dentistry, and how she's suffered. She expects that her dentist will listen and talk to her endlessly like her friends do. She's been rehearsing her story for weeks and is expecting the dentist to hang on every word. Anticipating her emotionally wrenching tale, she has a wad of tissues in her fist. She's ready to tell it all. Telling it all gets it off her chest and relieves her stress. She feels like she's been heard.

What does the stressed male dentist naturally want to do? Will listening and empathizing with Mrs. McBucks's problems relieve his stress? No way! In fact, the idea of listening to another "I hate dentists" story is like pounding another nail into the coffin. You see, over the course of the day our male dentist has been slowly withdrawing, talking less as the day wore on. In the morning he made superficial, clipped, small-talk with his patients and grunted at his staff. After lunch he's worse, feeling the effects of the morning and his big lunch. He's withdrawn and goes through the afternoon on automatic pilot, speaking just enough to get through the day.

Under these conditions, what will be the quality of the initial experience between Dr. Martian and Mrs. Mc Bucks? (Reread chapter five on communication skills—attitude, connecting, disclosure, and visual language.) What emotion will be behind his words—his attitude? Will he connect well with Mrs. McBucks, giving her his full attention? What will she be able to read in his eyes? How eager and willing will he be to disclose aspects of himself with which she can identify? How creative, colorful, and visual will his language be? If he is memorable, most likely what will Mrs. McBucks remember about him?

Most of the problems in dentistry stem from breakdowns in relationships among the dentists, staff members, and patients. *Men Are from Mars, Women Are from Venus*, a book originally intended to help men and women communicate in their romantic relationships and domestic arrangements, has much to offer in the dental office and case acceptance for complete dentistry.

CHAPTER 23

What's A Girl Like You Doing in a Place Like This?

Change is in the air, and the exclusive masculine model of dentistry is forever altered. A publication of the American Dental Association, *Distribution of Dentists in the United States by Region and State, 1998,* states that women dentists constitute 14 percent of active private practitioners and 33 percent of dentists in practice for ten or fewer years. In fact, nearly one-third of dentists who entered practice in the last ten years have been women.

Now that the rules have changed, women dentists have a golden opportunity to take advantage of trends in dentistry.

In particular, the trend toward elective procedures. Case acceptance for complete care and elective procedures are tailor-made for a woman's touch. One needn't have special "psychic powers" to predict that the next decade is going to spawn an awesome array of sophisticated, clinically excellent, successful women dentists. Twenty years ago, male dentists might have asked their female colleagues: "What's a girl like you doing in a place like this?" Hang around and they'll show us.

Not long ago, I approached a forty-something professional woman at a pool party and asked, "Would you feel comfortable going to a woman dentist?"

"Comfortable?" she shot back. "Are you kidding? I think I'd *prefer* a woman dentist."

"Why?"

"Because a woman instinctively knows what another woman needs, feels, and thinks. I'm old enough that I've got health concerns that a woman dentist my age would understand."

Male dentists can learn a lot from female dentists. I know I am treading on dangerous ground and running the risk of stereotyping men and women in our profession. However, after ten years of practice consultation, and especially through my collaboration with John Gray, Ph.D., on the video *Mars and Venus in the Dentist's Office*, I've had numerous occasions to observe and reflect on the differences between men and women in all areas of dental practice. Women are increasingly moving out of office jobs and the role of assistant and pursuing the education to take on that all-important seat next to the patient's chair as head of the practice. They bring a specific skill set and manner of behavior that is going to turn dentistry on its eyeteeth in the coming decade. And we men better pay attention.

The skills and attitudes generally associated with women—nurturing, listening, consensus building, caring—fit in perfectly with the kind of dentistry we all want and need to practice.

A Woman's Touch

A woman's touch is something you can see in her relationships, her appearance, and her skills. In general, women are good communicators; they ask questions, build rapport easily, are good listeners, enjoy giving compliments, and easily express their emotions. While admittedly, I'm generalizing, women look for harmony and are more likely to diminish the differences in expertise levels that exist between themselves and patients. Men are more interested in proving their expertise and are prone to show how much they know. In attempting to connect with a patient, a woman is less likely to use jargon than her male colleague, which means she more quickly removes barriers and builds trust.

Although this sounds superficial, women look good. In fact, because of their early conditioning, they have been working on looking good forever. This is not a trivial issue because *looking good* is the first step in creating the impression of *being good*.

In addition, women know how to ask for help without feeling weak. This is a major advantage in building a network of business advisors. Unlike so many male dentists who see themselves as "rugged individualists" who want to go it alone, a woman can create a support network, which ultimately, can help make the cash register ring.

A Woman's Intuition

A woman's intuition is revealed through her ability to be empathic. Women's capacity for empathy has earned them the societal stereotype of being kinder, softer, and gentler, which are powerful tools for a dentist. Empathy leads to understanding of what's going on inside the minds of patients and being able to anticipate another person's needs.

Jan, one of my wife's friends, said, "When I landed on the other side of forty, I got tired of men doctors. You have to draw them a picture."

Jan and millions of women like her are at the center of the target market for elective dental care (and other types of health care as well). Talk to these women and they will tell you that as they age, they're more likely to prefer the empathy demonstrated by female health care providers. Can a man show empathy? Of course, but it may not be—or seem—as "natural." It's like a bear riding a unicycle. The bear can do it, but it's not a natural action or skill. *Women know that empathy for another woman is instinctive.* That's hard to compete with, boys.

The Achilles' High Heel

While I am making broad and sweeping generalities let me add a warning based on some other typical traits we associate with the feminine. Because women can easily grow close to patients and staff, they are more vulnerable to sabotage and jealousy. Women's strengths can create their Achilles' heel. In her book

Women to Women, Judith Briles says women are more covert and indirect in unethical behavior, especially to other women. Briles says women are 30 percent more likely to behave unethically to other women than they are to men. What is the message women can take away from Briles' work? As John Gray says, "Be careful about being one of the girls with your staff and/or your women patients. Look to relationships outside the office to meet your personal needs."

It's a Matter of Time

It's only a matter of time before dentistry sees women emerge as clinical, management, and political leaders as influential as any male dentist has ever been. This has happened in other fields and it will happen within dentistry as well. Just look at athletics. In 1972, an amendment to an education bill established what we know as Title IX. The now famous Title IX mandates equal funding and promotion of women's athletic programs in schools receiving public funds. At the time, this proposition was quite controversial. High schools and universities were afraid that moving toward equal funding of men's and women's athletic programs would "dilute" the more important (read "revenue producing") men's sports programs. Most universities were not eager to achieve parity in athletic scholarships because they feared the money-making men's sports would suffer and quality would decrease.

To someone born after 1972, this whole discussion must seem bizarre. Hundreds of Olympic gold medals later, to name only one measure of success, we can see that in many cases, women's sports are sharing center stage with men. All women needed were opportunities and role models to show they could—in large numbers—become world-class athletes. In a similar way, once the law mandated that professional schools open the doors to men and women equally, women's enrollment immediately increased. I'm looking forward to the dramatic changes in dentistry that women are bringing as a result of equal opportunities.

The definition of success is changing. The workaholic, highly competitive, tooth jockey, big ego, fancy cars mentality of success is giving way to a kinder, gentler, and softer way. I believe that when the brass ring of success is viewed as having a healthy well-rounded lifestyle and quality relationships, it will be women who wear it.

CHAPTER 24

Look
Before You
Leap

Minimizing Dental Insurance

Successful case acceptance for complete dentistry kills two birds with one stone: You get to do some great dentistry and you *minimize the contamination of dental insurance*. If there's a secret to minimizing insurance it's this: *Become really good at what people want that insurance won't pay for*. I've structured this book to focus on case acceptance, and you'll be pleased to discover that the principles you've already learned are also the keys to minimizing dental insurance.

Frank, a dentist from Atlanta, called me and was brimming with excitement. "I'm going do it," he said. "I've made the decision to stop taking insurance assignment and no more prior authorizations. I'm getting dental insurance out of my hair once and for all."

I asked him why he thought that was a good thing to do. Frank sounded surprised by my question and said: "Hey, you say in your book, *Dentists: An Endangered Species*, that (and he quoted word for word,) 'no practitioner has ever built a reconstructive practice by relying on dental insurance.'"

He was right. I did say that, but before I could learn more about his situation, he continued: "Plus I've been to seminars and they say the best thing for dentists to do was to walk away from insurance all together. Cold turkey—just say no. I'm going for it."

"Frank, if I were you, I'd look before I leap. Do these seminars tell you what it's like to have patients leave your practice? Will they help you meet your payroll? Do these seminars base their recommendation on your specific needs or are the recommendations cookie-cutter solutions delivered safely from a podium?"

Frank was not pleased with my frankness. He was looking for the magic bullet to get his practice to the next level. He wanted to have a sophisticated restorative practice and he saw that other sophisticated restorative practices put dental insurance in the backseat. He figured if other high-end restorative practices had minimized dental insurance, then it must be the best thing for him. Right? Not always.

Frank, like many dentists, is confusing style with substance. He's like young high school athletes who get tattoos and wear their baseball caps sideways as they copy the look and style of professional superstar athletes. They hope that adopting a particular style will lead to improved performance.

> Dentists, like young athletes, would do more to improve their careers by copying the substance, not the style, of top practitioners.

Style Versus Substance

Look at the difference between the style and the substance of top practitioners. Style is the easiest to see, often is the most glamorous, and creates the most impact. But style varies and it changes with time—just about everything goes in and out of style. Style is also easy to emulate. Top practitioners have glamorous high-profile offices, in-office teaching institutes, celebrity patients, international travel, extraordinarily high fees, rigid financial arrangements, great affinity for new technology, and fancy marketing. These features of "style" represent the place to which top practitioners have evolved, but it's *not* where they started. All top practitioners started with substance.

Substance often goes unnoticed because it's not glamorous and is difficult to emulate. Substance does not change with time and the substance of top practitioners never varies. It includes three things: *excelling at providing what patients want, offering comprehensive treatment plans, and excellent relationship/communication skills.*

Substance enables style—not the other way around. If you want to minimize dental insurance, which is a feature of a particular style, in your practice, start with substance.

Minimizing Dental Insurance

Six steps to minimize dental insurance in your practice are presented below. The first three steps are based on substance; the last three relate to style:

Excel at Providing What Patients Want

To excel at doing what people want, combine technical excellence and mastery of the procedure with awareness that the patient's reason for wanting it is tied to its suitability. Suitability means four things: comfort, convenience, value, and improved appearance.

Comfort can mean many things. It may mean the absence of pain, but it can also mean the mental comfort patients experience when they know they will retain their teeth for their lifetime—lifetime strategies for dental health. Comfort can mean the ability to chew more easily. Comfort is a light touch. Comfort is an emotion that hovers over the many dental procedures and relationships, the emotional spectrum skills. Comfort settles in when patients feel safe, which is demonstrated through attitude and connection.

Convenience means realizing that patients' lives don't revolve around the dental office. For most people, the faster they get in and out and done with their care, the better they like it and the better they like you. They have more important things to do. Make it easy for patients to do business with you. Work with patients' schedules.

Value is surpassing patients' expectations, giving them a positive, unexpected experience, and giving them more than their money's worth. Value means staying within their budget and schedule.

Improved appearance is the best reminder of the comfort, convenience, and value the patient has experienced with you. Everybody wants to look better after your care than before. I've never met a patient who told me he or she wanted to look worse. Beauty sells.

Do you offer what people want or what you think they need? In other words, are you selling the *commodities* of dentistry. Do you sell pocket elimination surgeries, soft tissue treatments, crowns, laminates, or implants? If you do, then don't be surprised if patients don't want what you're selling. Know the difference between the procedure and its benefit: comfort, convenience, value, and improved appearance. Then communicate the benefit through attitude, connection, disclosure, visual language, the spectrum of appeal, and StorySelling, and let the procedure go along for the ride.

When you excel at treating target patients, your fees per case will increase to the level where dental insurance represents minimal value to the patient. Let's say the typical insurance limitation is 1200 dollars per year and your treatment plan is 2400 dollars. Insurance is 50 percent of this case. However, if your treatment plan is 10,000 dollars, then insurance is only 12 percent.

It's easier to convince someone to let the insurance company reimburse 12 percent of their case than 50 percent.

When you practice complete dentistry, dental insurance will not follow. When you provide lifetime strategies for dental health on older patients with significant dental breakdown, dental insurance will not follow. If you want to separate from the pull of insurance, go up.

Go up in the number of complete care patients you treat, and your fees will follow—you'll leave insurance behind.

Comprehensive Treatment Plan

Offer patients a lifetime strategy for dental health. Part of the substance of all great practitioners is their ability to recognize and provide complete care. Great cosmetic, implant, and restorative practitioners have strong skills in the fundamentals of occlusion, soft and hard tissue health, medical history, diagnosis, and restorative and preventative procedures. It is through understanding the comprehensive needs of the patient that great restorative, cosmetic, and implant practices grow.

Currently, it's in vogue to have a niche practice such as cosmetic, implant, or restorative. It's tempting to focus only on your niche, but when you do, the substance of a comprehensive approach can be crippled by the glitter of style. Become good at treating the whole mouth first; later, when you zero in on your niche, you're better positioned to recognize, treat, and/or refer dentistry to meet the patients' comprehensive needs.

A comprehensive approach in
diagnosis and treatment planning
is the substance that leads to
offering niche dentistry.

Perfect Relationship Skills

If you have excellent relationship skills, chances are great that you'll experience fulfillment in dentistry. Your relationships with your family, staff, patients, colleagues, and the public are the foundation of everything good in your practice. The greatest liabilities in dentistry are related to breakdown in relationships—divorce, malpractice, isolation, perfectionism, and addictions.

Relationship skills provide the staying power necessary to achieve top performance. Your technical expertise provides a good start, but most of your success will ultimately result from building and maintaining great relationships.

Your relationship with the patient
is the biggest bargaining chip in
the negotiation to minimize
insurance in your practice.

Substance is a prerequisite to minimizing dental insurance because we must give the patients a reason to accept our recommendations over those of their insurance company. The relationship with us must be more important to patients than their relationship with these companies. It's a trade: They get the benefit of our substance while we earn the right to ask them to deal with their insurance company on our terms, not the insurance company's. If we don't offer substance, we have nothing to offer in the trade. The next four steps to minimizing insurance relate to style.

Market Your Practice

To minimize insurance, you need an abundant number of mature target patients, those individuals who are more likely to be patients with comprehensive dental needs. Why should young adults who needs routine cleanings and minor procedures trade off their relationship with an insurance company? If the majority of your new patients are young, with most of their teeth, the substance of your practice has little to offer them.

Your marketing efforts should be focused on attracting new patients who are at least fifty years old. These patients have comprehensive needs and they place value on relationships with health care providers. When you try to minimize insurance, some patients will leave your practice. If you do not have an abundant flow of new patients, you'll be hesitant to follow your own rules and will give in out of necessity. For this reason, marketing programs should be ongoing.

Make Financial Arrangements with the Patient

The budget and financial arrangements involved in the lifetime strategy of a compelled target patient form the heart of your plan to minimize insurance. These patients are most likely to go along with your style of doing business.

Keep the financial arrangement simple. An arrangement that works well is to require one-third of the full fee at the beginning of care, one-third at an agreed upon midpoint, and the balance when the final restorations are placed. Once full payment has been made, then complete the insurance forms for the patient and direct assignment of benefits to the patient. Be sure to put these financial arrangements and insurance issues in writing and give the patients a signed original, and then put a copy in the record.

Convert Existing Patients Through Re-care

The hardest work in minimizing insurance is converting existing patients, especially those with minimal needs. The bad habit of accepting insurance has been established and the role of your team is to form new good habits. The first step in this process is to sell your team on the idea. If your team is not behind it, it will not work and you can forget the whole idea.

Next, create a list of benefits to patients that explains why pretreatment authorizations and assignment of benefits limit the range of care and lower the standards of care. These benefits are in the logical area of the Spectrum of Appeal. If you don't know these points or believe them, why should your patients?

Develop a consistent emotional spectrum message in your office. Tell the stories of patients who needed dentistry and objected to lack of insurance coverage but went ahead with the care, and are now living "happily ever after." Prepare printed materials that explain your position about insurance. Should you mail material to your patients and explain your new insurance position or should you discuss this in person? Both approaches can be successful. My clients' best results have come from explaining the new insurance rule in person, giving them printed materials, then instituting the new "insurance habit" on their next visit.

Put It in Writing

Here's a letter to patients about the benefits of minimizing dental insurance. It's available as a free download from my web site, www.paulhomoly.com.

Dear Patient,

Do the changes in the medical and dental insurance industry concern or confuse you? If so, you're not alone. Many of our patients are concerned about their dental insurance and how to get the most benefit.

To obtain the most benefit from your dental insurance, it's important to understand the *difference* between medical and dental insurance. Medical insurance is designed for *catastrophic events*—heart surgery, auto accidents, cancer treatment. Medical insurance carries high deductibles ($500-$1,000) you must pay out-of-pocket.

Dental insurance carries low deductibles ($50-$100), but offers *no coverage for catastrophic dental losses*—complete tooth loss, severe gum and bone diseases, complete dental breakdown. The irony is when patients need dental insurance the most, dental insurance offers very little.

Dental insurance has a low maximum annual benefit, usually less than $1,500. This means, that for patients with crippling dental problems, *dental insurance is no insurance at all*.

There are no tricks or loopholes to beat the dental insurance system. For patients with significant dental problems, to get the most from your dental insurance, follow these steps.

#1. Have a complete dental examination.

#2. Develop a lifetime plan for dental health.

#3. Implement your lifetime plan within a comfortable annual budget.

#4. File for dental insurance reimbursement when the budgeted dental care is completed.

#5. Continue to implement your lifetime plan each year, filing for reimbursement when that year's dental care is complete.

We can help you plan and budget your care so you get the most immediate relief from your dental problem and at the same time, maximize your insurance reimbursement. We've helped many patients get the most out of their dental insurance. We'll do the same for you.

Cordially,

Dr. Paul Homoly

The Rest of the Story

Dr. Frank from Atlanta was hoping that by adopting the style of established niche practices he would inherit their substance. It turns out that Frank practices in a competitive urban area, treats many young people with most of their teeth, does not market his practice, does not have a large number of new patients, and has no experience or advanced training with full mouth care. What is the probability that his patients will go along with his request to minimize the role of dental insurance in his practice? I'd say his chances are slim. Look before you leap.

My advice to Frank and to every dentist in his shoes is to develop substance before you impose your style. Like a professional athlete, get a solid game. Let your performance, your substance, do your talking. And after you're an MVP (Most Valuable Practitioner), let style become the icing on your cake.

CHAPTER 25

Going from Know
to
"Yes"

Who Do You Want to *Become?*

When I think back on all the dentists I've coached during the last ten years I see two distinct types. First we see dentists who study hard and make it a point to attend all the "right" courses. They leave these classes motivated, certain they have found the magic answer. However, in the end, they don't apply their new-found knowledge. And, like the miser millionaire who's afraid to let go of a nickel, they hoard what they know, and by not applying it, the information they hold in their hands doesn't do them or anyone else any good.

The second group of dentists looks beyond their vast collection of ideas and facts: They apply the information and transform it into results. They invest their knowledge in their practice and, hence, in all the lives that it touches. They understand the difference between knowing and doing, and when it comes to case acceptance, they understand how to go from "know" to "yes."

Dr. John Fish of Hildebran, North Carolina knows how to go from "know" to "yes." In the early eighties, right out of dental school, John associated in my practice. "From my first day in practice," John says, "I've enjoyed an insurance-free, fee-for-service practice. I could not pay a million dollars to replace the quality of the education and inspiration I've received."

John eventually bought my practice and today he's enjoying significant freedom and prosperity. I don't take credit for John's success. All I did was give John a good start.

This book will give you a good start. Here's how:

1. Study this book. Read it through, cover to cover, one time. Then reread it and use a highlighter to pull out key passages.

2. Watch the video presentation—it's a great tool to use at staff meetings.

3. Listen to the audio program several times while driving. You'll learn the dialogs just like you learn the words of songs when you listen to them many times.

4. Participate in Case Acceptance Coaching. Coaching is designed to support you and your team

in the new concepts and skills of case acceptance. The book, audio program, video presentation, and web site all are designed to be prerequisite materials for the coaching. They provide information; the coaching creates the skills. See www.paulhomoly for case acceptance coaching.

Confidence

I believe the passage from "know" to "yes" becomes easier as your confidence grows—confidence in your teachers and in yourself. Have confidence in this book. Every word comes from experience and is offered to help you practice the dentistry you love and prosper in the process.

Have confidence in yourself. Your life shrinks or expands in proportion to your level of self-confidence. We cannot grow our practices without first having the courage to grow ourselves. The best reason for success in dentistry is who we have to become to achieve it. Expect the best.

Dr. Paul Homoly
December 19, 2000